International Comparison of Health Care Data

Methodology development and application

International Comparison of Health Care Data

Methodology development and application

May 1999

Division Sociocultural Statistics
Department of Health and Welfare

Visiting address:
Prinses Beatrixlaan 428

Postal address:
P.O. Box 4000
2270 JM Voorburg

Telephone (..) 70 337 38 00
Fax: (..) 070 387 74 29

Visiting address:
Kloosterweg 1

Postal address:
P.O. Box 4481
6401 CZ Heerlen

Telephone (..) 45 570 60 00
Fax: (..) 45 572 74 40

Internet
http://www.cbs.nl

Kluwer Academic Publishers
Centraal Bureau voor de Statistiek

Authors: C.J.P.M. van Mosseveld
Statistical Researcher, Department of Health and Welfare,
Projectmanager (starting January 1st, 1998)
Tel.: .. - 31 70 337 5292 Fax: .. - 31 70 337 5979
e-mail: cmsd@cbs.nl

P. van Son
Project consultant, (until January 1st 1998)

Published by Kluwer Academic Publishers,
P.O. Box 17, 3300 AA Dordrecht, The Netherlands.

Sold and distributed in North, Central and South America
by Kluwer Academic Publishers,
101 Philip Drive, Norwell, MA 02061, U.S.A.

In all other countries, sold and distributed
by Kluwer Academic Publishers,
P.O. Box 322, 3300 AH Dordrecht, The Netherlands.

Printed on acid-free paper

The authors are fully responsible for the text in this report; the text does not necessarily correspond with the official point of view of Statistics Netherlands.

Contents

List of tables

List of figures and graphs

List of annexes

Preface

In 1994 the project "International Comparison of Health Care Data" was initiated by Statistics Netherlands at the request of the Ministry of Health, Welfare and Sports, which provided the necessary financial support.

The first phase of the project (1994–1995) focused on the intramural health care sector (see Literature no. 31). The second phase of the project (1996-1997) was devoted to extramural health care, prevention, other services and medical goods (see Literature no. 34). This report contains the description of the design, procedures and results of both phases.

Within the framework of the project the Ministry of Health, Welfare and Sports requested the collaboration for two special items, namely advanced medico-technological procedures (1996) and transport of patients (1997). Two distinct reports were produced on these subjects, based on inquiries of limited size (see Literature no's 34 and 35).

The realisation of this project would not have been possible without the valuable contributions from the participants in the network of experts from Belgium, Denmark, France, Germany and Switzerland, supplemented by participants from international organisations like OECD, WHO/Europe and EUROSTAT (see Annex 2.1).
Their contributions in terms of attending the yearly consultations and providing the data are gratefully acknowledged.

This work is only one step on the difficult road to improved international comparability of health care data. Reactions to the reports of the two phases showed great interest in the project. Further steps have been made by international organisations like Eurostat and OECD, based on the critical discussions of the approaches and results presented in the project.

Summary

In the Netherlands the organisation and financing of the health care system is currently undergoing a number of reforms. On many occasions the need has been felt to compare important national aspects of health care with those of other countries. In the Netherlands, as in other countries, international databases from e.g. OECD and WHO/Europe are being used for that purpose. Although the work done by these international organisations is highly valued. Their databases are not applicable to all desired aspects of international comparisons. Therefore the Ministry of Health, Welfare and Sports requested Statistics Netherlands (the international name for the Dutch central bureau of statistics) to start a project on the comparison of Dutch health care data with those of several neighbouring countries. Representatives from these countries (Belgium, Denmark, France, Germany and Switzerland) as well as from international organisations like OECD, WHO/EUR and EUROSTAT were invited to join a network of experts, in order to facilitate the exchange of ideas and information.

The aim of this project is to improve the comparability of a package of selected variables. The first phase of the project (1994 and 1995) were concentrated on statistics relating to intramural health care. Other health care sectors were examined in the second phase (1996 and 1997).

The project "International comparison of health care data" promotes a pragmatic approach to comparing the organisation and financing of the health care systems in the participating countries, leaving national definitions and methods of data collection intact.

Because of the different contents of health care systems, the activities or functions of health care as implemented by the providers have been taken as a starting point. A list of activities was sent to participants, and they were requested to indicate which activities are performed by which health care provisions. Based on the information received, a set of provisions was constructed which was used in the process of determining the boundaries of the health care systems of the participating countries.

The boundaries of care were defined more precisely during the process of bilateral comparisons which took the Dutch health care system as its starting point and resulted in five distinct bilateral comparable packages.

In the next step the possibilities were examined of creating a multilateral comparison, named the Common Comparable Package (CCP), based on the results of the five bilateral comparisons. The CCP of health care for the participating countries was constructed by means of additions, deductions and reshuffling of provisions. This CCP can be used as a reference, an instrument for international comparison.

This volume contains the results Phase I dealing with Intramural health care (see literature no. 33) and of Phase II dealing with the categories of Extramural health care, Preventive health care, Medical goods and Other services, (see literature no. 36). Results of Phase I on Intramural health care have been revised and updated in Phase II.

Below the results of the process of constructing a Common Comparable Package on Health are summarised.

Table 1
Summary of health care expenditures, 1994

	Netherlands	Germany	Switzerland	Belgium
Year 1994				
Expenditures: OECD Health Data Bank 1997				
Expenditures in % of GDP	8.8	10.3	9.6	8.1
Expenditures per capita (US $)	1,923	2,581	3,496	1,845
Expenditures per capita (ECU)	1,621	2,178	2,956	1,557
Expenditures: Common Comparable Packages				
Expenditures in % of GDP	7.9	9.7	9.1	7.3
Expenditures per capita (US $)	1,724	2,459	3,312	1,644
Expenditures per capita (ECU)	1,453	2,069	2,800	1,387

The expenditures on health care as a percentage of Gross Domestic Product range in the CCP-approach from 7.2 percent (Denmark 1995) to 10.4 percent (France 1995). The OECD calculating these same shares presents a range from 6.4 percent (in Denmark 1995) to 10.3 percent (for Germany in 1994).

The percentages spent on health in the CCP-approach differ from those presented by the OECD. In some cases like Denmark, France and Belgium these percentages are higher; in other cases like the Netherlands, Germany and Switzerland they are lower. More important is that the relative differences between the countries in the CCP-approach are generally smaller than in the OECD data. This means that the uniformed contents of the package in the CCP is confirmed by raw data for the participating countries.

Table 1 (end)
Summary of health care expenditures, 1995

	Netherlands	Denmark	France	Switzerland	Belgium
Year 1995					
Expenditures: OECD Health Data Bank 1997					
Expenditures in % of GDP	8.8	6.4	9.9	9.8	8.0
Expenditures per capita (US $)	2,232	2,108	2,616	4,210	2,126
Expenditures per capita (ECU)	1,711	1,611	1,999	3,205	1,627
Expenditures: Common Comparable Packages					
Expenditures in % of GDP	7.9	7.2	10.4	9.2	7.4
Expenditures per capita (US $)	2,016	2,390	2,754	3,942	1,968
Expenditures per capita (ECU)	1,546	1,825	2,104	3,001	1,504

In the table above the expenditures on health care measured in US dollars per capita are presented as well. In the CCP-approach the data range from $ 1,644 in Belgium (1994) to $ 3,942 in Switzerland (1995). In the OECD data set the lowest expenditures per capita are seen for Belgium ($ 1,857) in 1994; the highest in Switzerland for 1995 ($ 4,210).

1. Introduction

Every nation has built up a structure of organising and financing of health care based on historical conditions and national concepts of social solidarity and justice. Nowadays these national concepts receive mighty impulses from international panels. Governments are challenged to solve their health care policy problems against the background of international philosophies and programmes like the new Health for All programme of the World Health Organisation and other international organisations like the OECD and the European Union. The latter has entered the field of public health by the Maastricht treaty in 1992. Like WHO and OECD did before the EU paid attention to the development of information systems to support the policy development in this field.

It may be clear, that these developments have a long-term perspective. Reaching consensus on common conceptual frameworks as a solid base for practically applicable information systems must follow time-consuming procedures.

Meanwhile countries are confronted with the short-term need to reform their health care systems under the increasing pressure of rising costs. At the same time their cost containment policies should not affect accessibility, quality and solidarity. International orientation on policy instruments takes place from the viewpoint, that if these policy instruments are successful in one country, they might also be successful in other countries.

Comparing results of different ways of organisation of health care and the use of specific instruments to guarantee the fair distribution of the benefits of the system among the population requires a certain transparency of the national health care systems. This transparency should be provided by the availability of valid comparable data.

Therefore the Ministry of Health, Welfare and Sports requested Statistics Netherlands (the international name for the Dutch central bureau of statistics) to start a project on the comparison of Dutch health care data with those of a selected number of countries: Denmark, Germany, Switzerland, France and Belgium.

Experts from these countries were invited to form a network for information and consultation. Representatives from WHO/EUR, OECD and EUROSTAT also participated in this network.

The project aimed at the improvement of the comparability of a package of selected variables. These variables refer to the production function of health care supply, consumption, cost and financing. This goal has been reached only partially. Data on supply, consumption and especially manpower were not available in sufficient quality and quantity.

The first phase of the project (1994–1995) concentrated on statistics relating to intramural (in-patient) health care. A great deal of attention was paid to methodology development. In the second phase (1996–1997) the approach, that had been developed in the first phase, was applied to extramural care (outpatient care), preventive health care, medical goods and other services. The field described in Phase II can be characterised by an enormous diversity of activities and heterogeneity of functions, in contrast to the relative uniformity of the field described in Phase I of the project on Intramural health care on which updated data are presented in this publication as well.

The project did not aim at the development of a set of definitions on common concepts and procedures. This would take too much time and in the last instance would require changes and adaptations of national health information systems. Leaving intact national definitions insight was gained by so called "country profiles", brief and general overviews of the national health care systems involved and by a set of descriptions of provisions in operational terms.

2. Process

2.1 *Aims and objectives*

The overall aim of this project is to improve the international comparability of health care data. In order to benefit more from the experiences with changing health care policies in other countries, the Dutch authorities want to compare their system with those in other countries. For this comparison a package was assembled containing selected variables on supply (provisions and manpower), consumption, and the costs and financing of health care. It should be stressed that the project focuses on broad categories of care and sets of variables, i.e. macro-level comparability and statistical data, not on figures for administrative purposes.

Within the general framework concrete objectives have been formulated for improvement of international comparability of health care data. These objectives are:

- the collection of comparable data on supply (provisions, manpower), consumption an cost of Intamural health care
- the collection of comparable data on costs and financing of extramural health care, preventive health care, medical goods and other services;
- determination of the boundaries of health care;
- improving the methodology for international comparison;
- description and comparison of the health care systems of the participating countries by means of a reference model;
- development of keys for conversions to be used in comparison.

In phase II (more than in phase I) problems showed up with regard to the availability of data on supply, consumption and manpower. Therefore in Phase II attention was focused on expenditures and financing. In this book, combining the results of the two phases, only limited attention is given to non-financial data.

Leading papers, written by some members of the network (Dr. M. Schneider, Dr. S. Sandier, J.-P. Poullier and C.J.P.M. van Mosseveld/J.M. Smit), were the first explorations of the fields of supply, consumption, manpower and as well helped to built the general approach. These leading papers have been bundled separately in an annex (Annex 2.5).

2.2 *Network of experts*

One important element of this project is the functioning of a network of experts. Statistics Netherlands has had very good results with this approach on many occasions as in the development of common methods and instruments for Health

Interview Surveys. This interactive approach is characterised by the exchange of information in writing (e.g. by leading papers) and other means and intensive consultation sessions of the network members as strong incentives for progress.

By emphasising the exchange of information the network facilitated the production of the "country profiles" (see chapters 3 through 8).

Moreover, the members of the network suggested relevant aspects of work to be done, like:

- emphasising the need for definitions;
- mutual information on relevant developments concerning information policy with regard to health care;
- exploration of opportunities of satellite accounts for international comparison;
- information on the development of the German health report system and its possible contribution to international comparison of health care data;
- discussion on the use of PPP (Purchasing Power Parity) in international comparison of health care data;
- suggestions for conclusions and recommendations on future work.

For practical reasons an initial choice was made for experts from neighbouring countries (Belgium, Denmark, Germany, Switzerland and France). Representatives of international organisations (OECD, WHO, Eurostat) were also invited to participate (see Annex 2.1).

Consultations took place in Voorburg on 21–23 September 1994, 4–6 October 1995, November 18–19 1996 and finally on November 4–5 1997.

2.3 *General approach*

The project "International comparison of health care data" advocates a pragmatic approach to comparing the organisation and financing of the health care systems in the participating countries.

The starting point for this approach is the description of health care used by Statistics Netherlands.

Health care concerns the supply of goods and services in the area of medical, paramedical and nursing care:

- *provided for human beings suffering from diseases, physical and/or mental disabilities or limitations;*
- *related to prevention, diagnostics, treatment and nursing/caring;*
- *provided by trained experts and/or companies (or parts of companies) set up for this purpose.*

Every country has its own views on the description, institutionalisation and organisation of health care, usually the outcome of a long history of government decisions to solve imminent problems. National health care provisions are thus made to measure, in tune with feelings of social justice among the population and with the organisation and functioning of other institutions in society. Against this historical background it is understandable that health care systems have different contents, different organisational forms and different financial sources.

Because of the different contents of health care systems, within the framework of the project attention was paid first to the activities or functions of health care as implemented by the providers. Participants were sent an activity list with the quest to indicate which activities are performed by which health care provisions. The returned lists provided basic information for an overview of health care provisions: data on the existence of provisions and related expenditures and financing sources.

Thus an overall insight has been obtained into the boundaries of the health care systems of the participating countries, according to the following steps (See Annex 2.2: List of activities and Annex 2.3: Boundaries/Provisions):

Activities → Provisions → Costs → Financial sources

The boundaries of care were defined more precisely during the process of bilateral comparisons which took the Dutch health care system as a starting point (see figure 2.1).

Figure 2.1: Bilateral Comparison

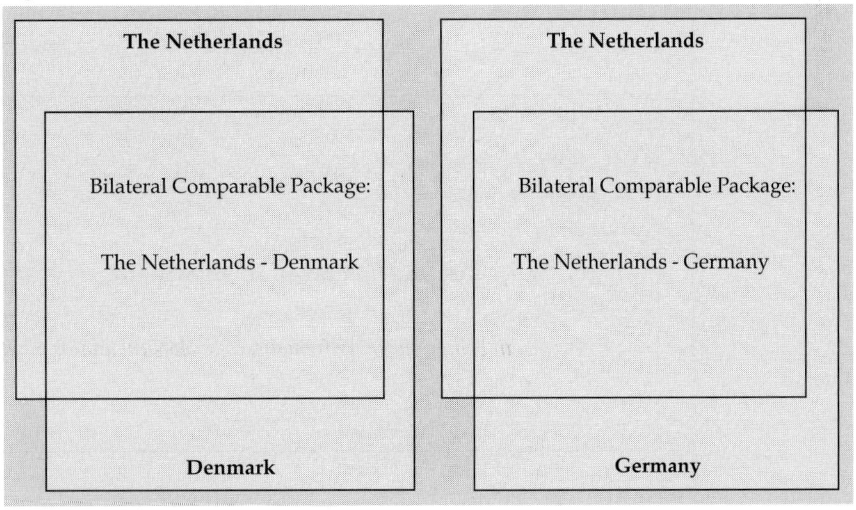

The next step examined the possibilities of creating a Common Comparable Package (CCP) of health care, based on the results of the bilateral comparisons (see figure 2.2).

Figure 2.2: Towards a Common Comparable Package

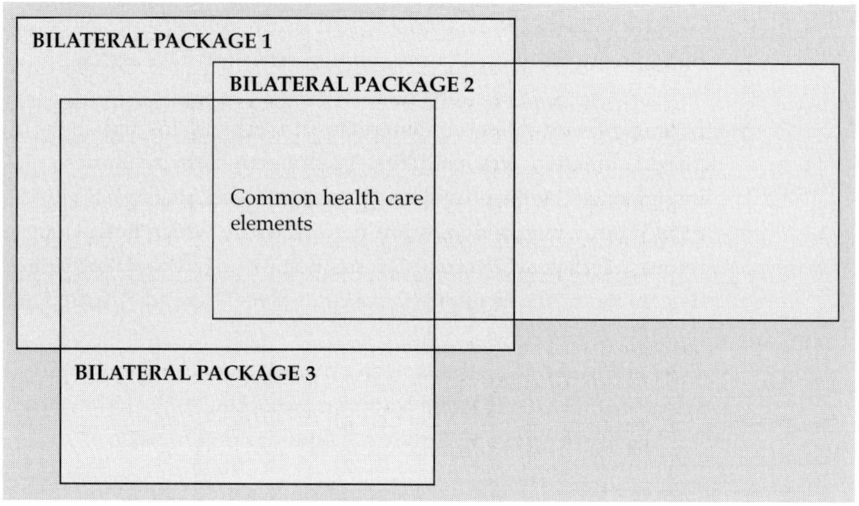

By means of additions, deductions and reshuffling of provisions, the CCP of health care for the participating countries was constructed. This CCP (figure 2.3) can be used as a reference, a common concept (instrument) for international comparison.

Figure 2.3: The Common Comparable Package

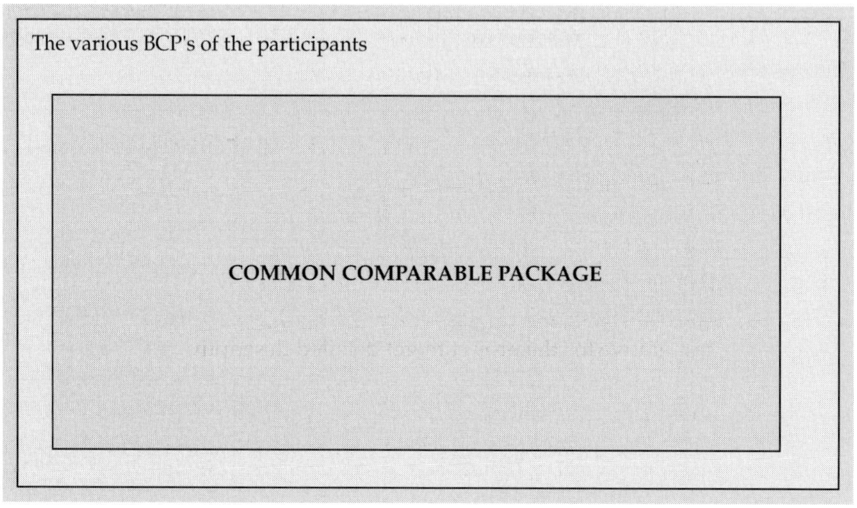

2.4 *Description of the process*

The data collection process consisted of the following steps:

a. *List of operational definitions* (see Annex 2.4)
Right from the very beginning of the project, definitions of activities and services in health care were considered crucial. A provisional inventory of definitions was produced. As the construction of a system of definitions used in health care soon proved to be too time consuming, an operational list, based on CBS definitions, was drawn up to help participants understand the nature of Dutch health care provisions. During the process this set of operational definitions was expanded and improved according to the need felt at that moment, but not with the intention to develop an exhaustive, well-structured and final set of definitions.

b. *List of activities* (see Annex 2.2)
Based on an analysis of activities performed in health care (together with the country profiles), a list of activities was drawn up (see Annex 2.2). The aim was to get insight into which activities are performed by which provisions.

c. *List of provisions* (see Annex 2.3)
Based on the response received to the list of activities, a list of provisions was compiled consisting of all health care provisions indicated by participants.

d. *Matrices*
The list of health care provisions served as the core for two questionnaires in the form of matrices. The first dealt with the existence of provisions in the participating countries their inclusion in the health care sector or other sectors. The information received (especially information about expenditure) formed the basis for the determination of boundaries of care. The second matrix dealt with the financial sources of the provisions.

Below the method used in this project and the model developed accordingly is described in more detail.

2.4.1 *Description of the method*

Knowing that comparability can only be obtained by eliminating differences, and differences can only be eliminated by having information on these differences, it was imperative for the project to get detailed descriptive information on the health care systems of the participating countries.
The descriptive information that was supplied at the request of Statistics Netherlands resulted in the country profiles, a selected description of the functioning of the health care system.

It is known that knowledge of the system alone is not enough to create comparison. Knowing how health care is organised, what actors or providers are involved is necessary but not sufficient. It is common knowledge that separate activities are supplied in different combinations in various countries. And knowledge of the combinations of activities and providers is essential. So an extensive list of activities was created, originating in the country profiles and supplemented by information from literature. Activities are the actions in the health care field that can be separately distinguished. Actors or providers are the nationally defined clusters of activities that are able to supply the data.

This list of activities was sent to the participants with the request to supply all the actors/providers of health care performing those activities. This resulted in a country specific set of activities and their providers.
All these country specific lists of providers made it possible to create one list of providers.

Figure 2.4: Method

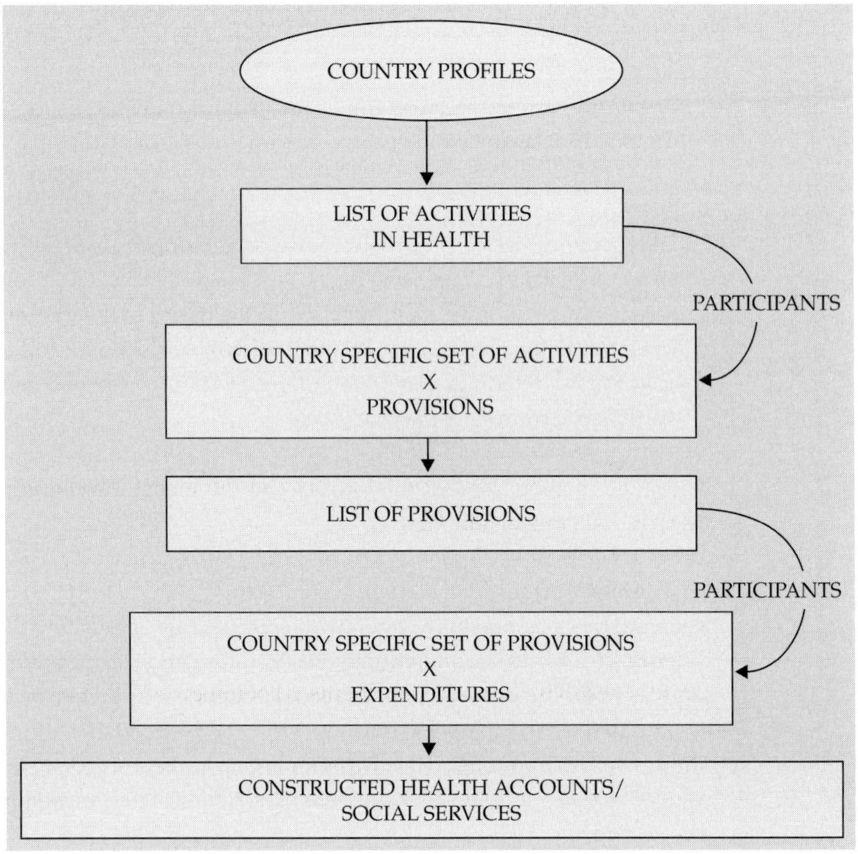

Next, information on providers and corresponding expenditures was needed. So this list of provisions were sent to the countries to specify which provisions are present in their (health or national) accounts, and the expenditures on these provisions.

Returned were country specific sets of provisions with amounts of expenditures or costs. Every participant was asked to add annotations, remarks and questions to this list. These lists made it possible to construct a health account for every country containing the providers of health care and their expenditures.

2.4.2 *Description of the model*

Figure 2.5: Towards a theoretical model

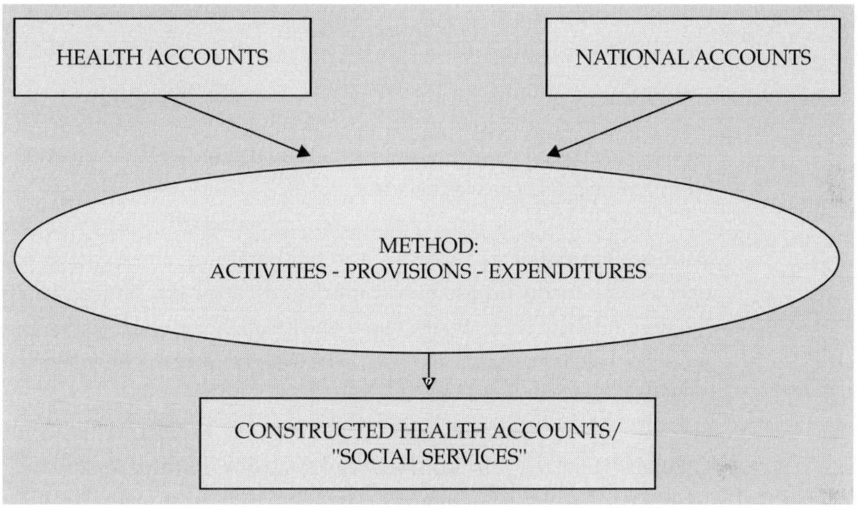

Figure 2.5 presents the summary of the approach followed, the method used in the project. The core theme of the project was the notion that expenditures can only be obtained at the provider level in the health care system; that these providers are different in various countries, but that a lot of activities in the health care field are the same whatever the system used.

Whether or not the data of the countries were collected in the health accounts or the sector of health in the national accounts is not important. The goal of neither system is international comparability, but a.o. completeness given different starting points. The method of activities linking to providers and providers linking to expenditures offered the possibility to construct a health account. This constructed health account could also include some services that are listed as welfare services or social services.

Figure 2.6: Towards a Bilateral Comparable Package (BCP)

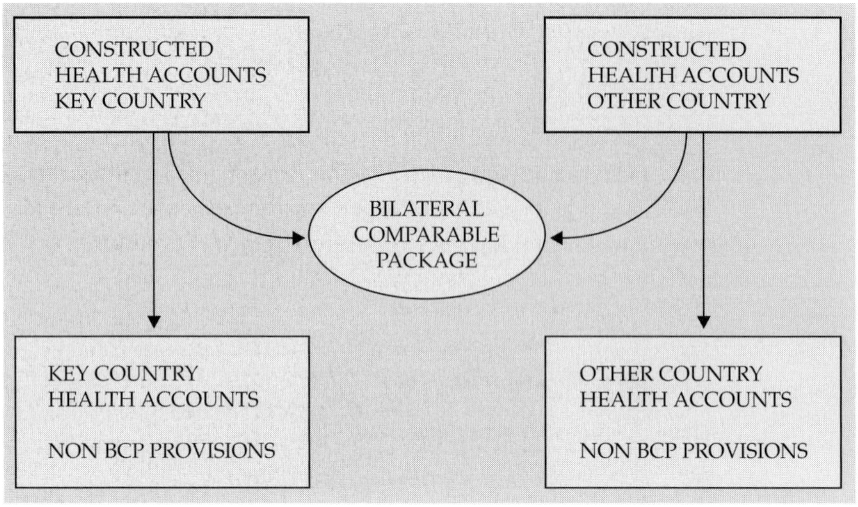

At least one step between the information at hand and the creation of multilateral comparable packages was necessary.

Because the goal of this exercise was comparability, the idea was launched to limit every comparison to just two countries. Because the project was initiated in the Netherlands and we knew best how, the Dutch health care system is the key country in every comparison. This first part of the process resulted in five bilateral comparisons.

Comparing the systems of two countries, using all the data at hand, but especially the data on the activities gave the possibility to separate every health account in three parts: one on a set of provisions (containing a comparable cluster of activities) in both countries, and two other sets of provisions not available in the Netherlands and the other country (the so-called non Bilateral Packages).

The set of providers in both countries is the so-called Bilateral Comparable Package. If for any reason a comparison of just two countries is needed, this BCP-approach is the solution.

Having six countries in the project and selecting one country to be the key country resulted in five distinct Bilateral Packages. Although each pair of results was comparable, the five Bilateral Packages were not. The package of the key country was different in every bilateral comparison. A multilateral comparable package was needed, in which all the bilateral packages were transformed to one multilateral comparable package, the so-called Common Comparable Package.

Figure 2.7: Towards a Common Comparable Package (CCP)

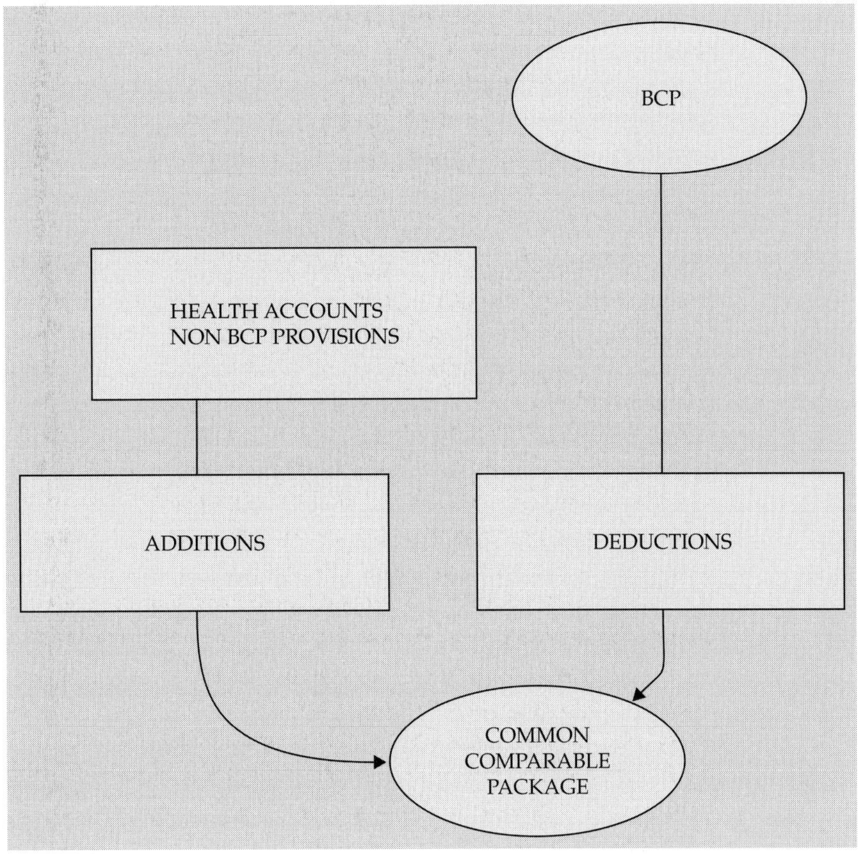

One way to solve this problem is to create multilateral comparison by excluding every provision or part of it that was not present in every country. The consequence of this approach would have been that each inclusion of a new country would limit the contents of the comparable package, ultimately resulting in a very thin comparable package.

Another approach is to include every provision of any of the participants constructed Bilateral Package. This approach could lead to the opposite; a continuous expanding comparable set.

So a different approach was taken. In this approach those provisions are included that are listed either in the Bilateral Packages or in the non Bilateral Packages as long as the activities of these provisions can be fitted into the general notion of health care. As a consequence some additions and deductions were necessary, but only in a limited number of cases. Another consequence is that a rather stable package could be constructed, that does not need to change when a country is included or excluded.

Figure 2.8: Completed model

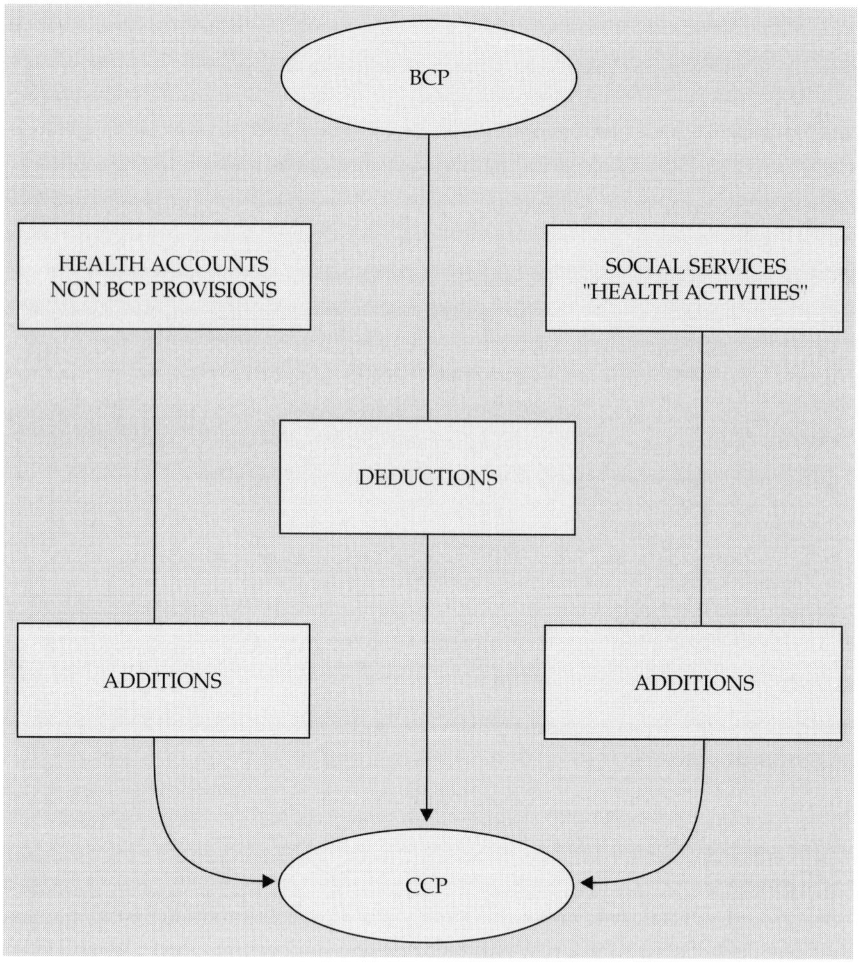

The general notion of being part of the health accounts had one problem, namely that some provisions had to be added that were not part of the health accounts in some country but part of the social sector.

The last problem to be solved concerned calculations of parts of provisions or sets of activities, although present in any country, for which no data could be supplied separately. Sometimes it concerned a reshuffling of expenditures from one sector to another sector inside the health accounts. In other cases the amount of expenditures had to be calculated as an addition to the CCP. Of course in creating a common comparable package some provisions are eliminated from the bilateral comparisons because they are not providing health activities, in spite of the fact that in some countries these provisions and their activities are included in the health accounts.

Figure 2.9: Method & Completed model

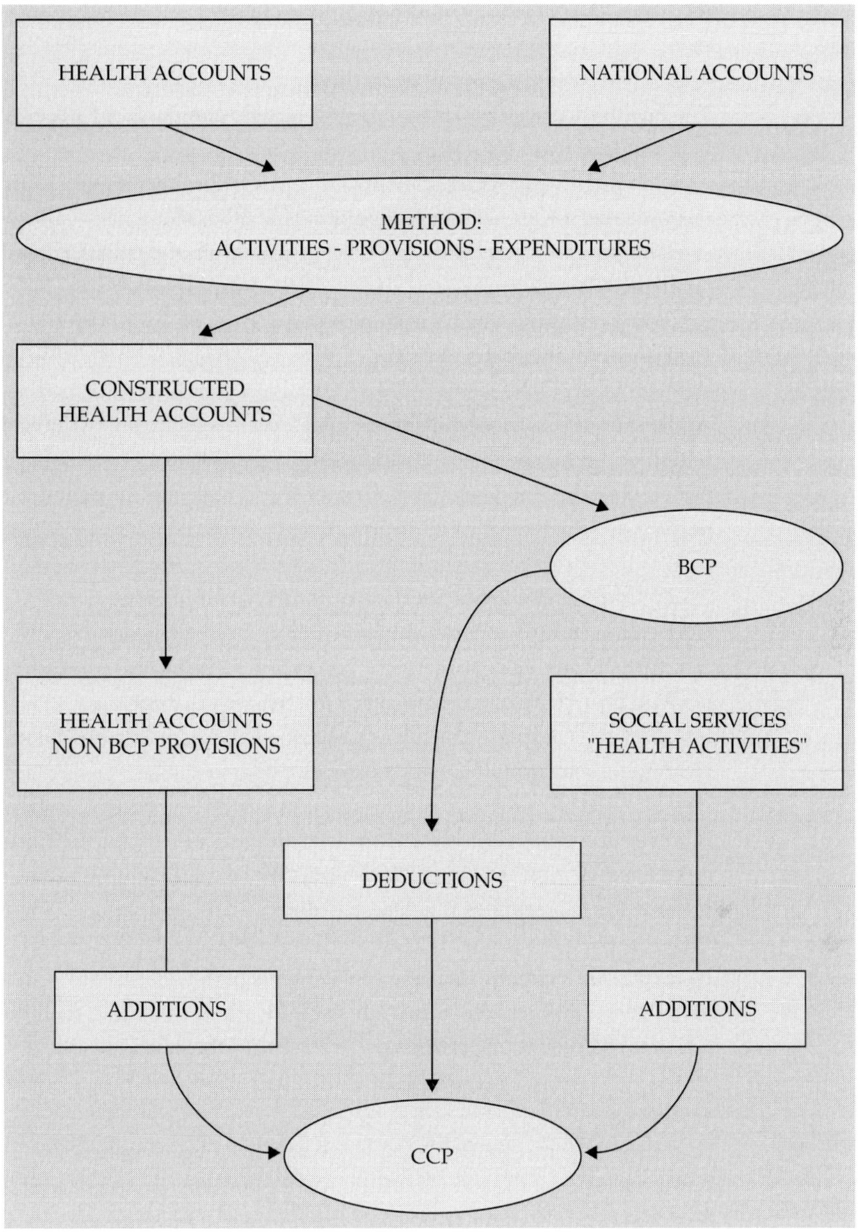

This last figure (figure 2.9) on the method and model of the CCP presents the complete picture. Starting with the health or national accounts, using the method to reach a bilateral package, using all the bilateral packages, adding and deducting some provisions or parts of provisions ultimately leads to a common comparable package.

2.5 *Methodological remarks*

2.5.1 *The direct comparison method*

The health care systems of two countries were compared by observing the content of both health care packages:

- setting apart equal elements in a comparable package of goods and services;
- observing differences or particularities of other elements;
- estimating the consequences of these differences or particularities in, for example, financial terms;
- adding or subtracting related amounts to/from the expenditures of the health care systems under observation.

At the start of this procedure at national level it is important to have determined the boundaries of the health care systems and to have listed the elements included. Costs are always the financial translation of these elements in action and financing is defined as the division of costs according to financial resource.

2.5.2 *Conversion or the method of indirect comparison*

Conversion simply means the translation from one standard to another – for example: inches to centimetres – according to standard computing rules. In the present project, conversion is used in this sense, monetary exchange rates, for instance, for comparing health care costs. Where such conversion standards are lacking, references will have to be developed.

But even if we have such standards at our disposal, supplementary activities will be needed to combine them with non-standard elements to achieve an accurate comparison, covering as much as possible.

If stable relationships exist between elements of the health care system, then "keys" are of great importance. If no such stable relationships exist, then the best possible estimates can serve our purposes. To start with the latter:

a. Estimates

Lacking data for a simple variable, the value can be estimated; not as a wild guess, but as the result of the trained intuition of e.g. an experienced statistician. In this way, based on considerations of possible minimum and maximum limits, the amount for over the counter medicines in the Netherlands has been estimated at a value of 250 millions guilders a year (1994).

b. Keys

A more solid estimate can be reached by using "keys", relative fixed value indicators expressing a more or less constant relationship between part and total. For example:

costs of outpatient departments in Dutch hospitals. These costs cannot be separated from total hospital costs. After calculations some years ago the National Hospital Institute attributed 40% of the costs to nursing and nursing care, 30% to clinical diagnostics and treatment and another 30% to outpatient diagnostics and treatment. Once these more or less constant percentages were fixed, they are used as "keys" until new calculations are done. Keys are important at many moments in the process of comparison, where sufficient specifications cannot be made. Because the costs of outpatient care in German hospitals are negligible, 30% of the costs of Dutch hospitals should be subtracted before comparing the costs of Dutch and German hospitals.

c. References

References or standards can be based on theoretical outcomes or general consensus (e.g. describing a standard hospital), but in this context a reference can be based on the pragmatic, empirical approach of the Common Comparable Package: a package of care components, present in the health care system of the participating countries. The advantages of such empirically developed references are clear:

- data are available, at least partially, and it may be expected that the quality can be improved;
- functional transparency; in principle the provisions involved are known and, consequently, the activities performed by these provisions.

2.5.3 *Definitions*

The project itself does not aim to develop common concepts and procedures, which would eventually require changes and adaptations of national information systems.

Of course it was necessary to define a number of health care provisions in operational terms. The limitations of this approach with regard to conceptualisation are clear. Nevertheless, what has been done in this field, together with notions of consensus among participants, was felt to be feasible and manageable in this phase.

In the communication with participants this pragmatic approach has provoked discussions on common concepts and common theoretical frameworks, which are seen as indispensable for international comparison.

Further refinement necessary for this project will also require attention for definitions and the development of a logical structure in which they will fit. More attention for definitions does not mean that national concepts and definitions are adapted or changed. What is meant is an intrinsic characterisation of what must be defined. A logical structure is an ordering of concepts and definitions from general categories to subcategories in which every relevant entity in the field of health care can be classified.

2.5.4 *Classifications*

In the course of the project several attempts were made to develop useful classifications of health care services. Ultimately the following classification was used in the questionnaires: intramural care, extramural care, preventive care, medical goods, subdivided into pharmaceutical and therapeutical appliances and other services. This classification was based on an analysis of activities and provisions in the field of health care.

3. Country profile: The Netherlands

3.1 Introduction

The exchange of information in the network of experts facilitated the production of the "country profiles", which are meant to provide:

- a quick introduction to the organisation and administration of the health care systems of the participating countries;
- an exploration of the boundaries of the health care system;
- a preliminary determination of place and functions of health care;
- an overview of the main policy developments;
- a contribution to transparency, a necessary condition for international comparison.

The country profiles contain information on health care administration, financing, policy dvelopments and the organisation of health care. This information was brought together in the two phases of the project "international comparison of health care data".

In the first phase (1994–1995) the boundaries of the national health care systems were explored. Also general characteristics of health care administration, financing, policy developments and health care organisation were described.

Detailed quantative data became available on intramural health care. The expression "ïntramural health care" proved to be a typically Dutch one. Intramural health care is by and large equal to in-patient health care or stationary care. The description used (see Annex 2.4) is health care for patients formally admitted for a period of more than 24 hours and/or institutionalised treatment for a substantial part of the day (or night).

In the second phase of the project (1996–1997) more detailed data were collected on extramural care, preventive health care, medical goods and other services. Also attention was paid to an update of the determination of the boundaries of national health care systems.

Also the expression "extramural health care" proved to be a typically Dutch one. Extramural health care is described as health care provided on a non-residential basis by medical and paramedical professionals or by specialised organisations in home care or home nursing (for a complete description see Annex 2.4).

At the start of the project the intention was to provide country profiles for all the sectors of care described in this report. This goal was not reached. Especially

information on the topic of "other services" is lacking. To a lesser extent the same holds true for the topic of "medical goods".

3.2 *Aspects of general administration of health care*

Although under the national constitution Dutch government is obliged to take measures for the advancement of public health, the health care system is based on a complex division of responsibilities, in which the government and government institutions, but also private organisations and independent professionals and their associations are allocated their own share of responsibilities.

Since 1988 this system has been undergoing rapid transformations, with the traditional relationships developing towards a more market-oriented health care system, in which parties like providers of care, financers and consumers are acting in new roles. The government will retain overall responsibility, but will act more from a background position. At the moment, however, government plays an active role in directing the necessary reforms and regulating the new relationships between parties in the field of health care. In the present situation the Minister of Health, Welfare and Sport has overall responsibility for the health services and the power to issue orders, guidelines and instructions, in accordance with acts of Parliament. He holds a key position in respect of health care standards, planning and construction, training and remuneration of health care staff. He also determines the level of income-dependent contributions to be paid to the various statutory insurance funds and the benefits to be provided. The Health Inspectorate, attached to the Ministry, supervises compliance with health care standards. A number of advisory bodies, of which the most important are the National Council of Public Health and the Health Insurance Council, also fulfil an important forum function for the many private organisations active in the field of health care.

Administrative and executive responsibility at regional and local level lies with the twelve provinces (regional facility planning) and the well over 700 municipalities (preventive services).

3.3 *Financing of health care*

Data on the financing of health care in the Netherlands can hardly be compared from year to year without extensive explanations. There are two reasons for this:

a. Up to 1988 the Ministry of Welfare, Health and Culture annually published the "Financial Survey of Health Care" as an Annex to the budget. From 1989 the title of this publication was changed to "Financial Survey of Care", as an expression of the policy target to integrate health and social care, which were brought together in the sector "care".
   This political line was not followed by Statistics Netherlands, which maintained

its list of health care provisions on behalf of the statistics "cost and financing of health care". That is why in the "Financial Survey of Care" the total expenditure on care was 55.8 thousand million guilders in 1992, while Statistics Netherlands computed 47.9 thousand million guilders, limited to health care in he strict sense. Authors dealing with comparison of health care data and continuing to rely on the "Financial Survey" risk using an incorrect total and numerator and as well as an incorrect share of general taxation, because especially with regard to provisions in the social care sector government subsidies dominate. For example, in publications based on the "Financial Survey" general taxation contributes up to 10%, in publications of Statistics Netherlands only 5%.

b. Within the framework of organisational and financing reforms in health care, some provisions (e.g. pharmaceuticals) have been brought under the Exceptional Medical Expenses Act. This meant the elimination of these provisions from the packages of the private insurance companies, because the Act mentioned applies to every citizen. This explains the increase of social security as financial source in the data 1991–1992 in the following table, accompanied by a decrease of the addition of individual payments/private insurance.

Table 3.1
The Netherlands: Financial sources, 1991, 1992 (percentages of total)

	Financial Survey of Care		Cost & Financing of Care	
	1991	1992	1991	1992
General taxation	10.4	10.2	5	5
Social security	64.5	67.6	68	72
Individual payments	8.5	8.0	27 [2]	23 [1]
Private insurance	16.6	14.2		
Total	100.0	100.0	100	100

[1] Including private insurance.

3.4 *Insurance structure*

The sickness insurance system in the Netherlands is built on three pillars: the Exceptional Medical Expenses Act (AWBZ), the Sickness Fund Act (ZFW) and private insurance.

The Exceptional Medical Expenses Act provides compulsory insurance for all residents, originally covering the high costs of long-term care e.g. hospital stays of longer than one year, stays in nursing homes, institutions for the physically and mentally handicapped. In recent years other provisions have become part of the AWBZ package e.g. ambulatory mental care, pharmaceuticals and therapeutical appliances, audiological care, genetic counselling and preventive care like vaccinations and the detection of congenital metabolism disorders. The contribution to the AWBZ is income related and consists of a fixed percentage (in 1994: 8.55%) of income under the first bracket of taxation. The administration of benefits is handled by the patient's insurer, sickness fund or private insurance.

Other costs of health care are covered either by the sickness funds (under the Sickness Fund Act), or by private insurance. The sickness funds are compulsory for employees with an income below a yearly fixed level (58,100 guilders per year on 1-1-1994) and social security benificiaries (including the elderly). 61% of the population is covered under this scheme. Civil servants employed by provincial and municipal governments are covered by a compulsory insurance scheme (6% of the population), which is similar to a private insurance.

The contributions to the sickness funds are paid by employers (in 1994 5.15% of the employee's gross wage) and by the employees (in 1994 1.2% of their gross wage). Moreover a nominal contribution per insured person is paid to the insurer (fl. 185 per year per adult; half this amount per child with a maximum of two children). The level of contributions is fixed by the government yearly. For a small additional amount the sickness funds offer their insured a voluntarily supplementary insurance for provisions such as dentures and spectacles.

There is no compulsory insurance for the self-employed and salaried people with wages above the cut-off level. About 33% of the population are privately insured with one of the many private insurance companies. Premiums are nominal and are to some extent risk-related. The premium is paid directly to the private insurance company. Generally privately insured often can select the composition of their "insurance package" and are free to choose a fixed amount as deductibles in return for premium reduction.

3.4.1 *Sickness fund benefits*

The Exceptional Medical Expenses Act (AWBZ) covers the costs of extended hospital stay (more than one year), home care, nursing homes, out-patient and intramural psychiatric care, care for the physically and mentally handicapped, pharmaceuticals, therapeutic appliances, genetic counselling and audiological services.

The sickness fund insurance covers medical care (general practitioners, out-patient specialists), physiotherapy, speech therapy, midwifery, dental care, short stay and day care in hospitals, patient transport and maternity care. AWBZ and sickness fund benefits are provided in kind. Private insurance companies mostly reimburse the costs of care to their clients within the boundaries of the chosen "package" of the insurance.

3.4.2 *Cost sharing*

At the moment co-payments are levied under the sickness fund scheme for maternity care (intramural and extramural), for dental provisions like dentures, crowns and false teeth, and for transportation of patients except transport by ambulance. Other forms of co-payments concern clinical plastic surgery, psychotherapy, physiotherapy, home care and therapeutic appliances. Spectacle lenses are partially reimbursed.

Drugs are free at fixed prices. This means that the average in a group of equal therapeutic value determines the price. If more expensive drugs are chosen the patient pays the difference. Under the AWBZ scheme co-payments are required during stay in institutions. Under private insurances individual payments depend on the composition of the chosen insurance package.

3.5 *Fee and salary structure*

Sickness funds pay capitation fees to general practitioners. The full tariff applies for the first 1600 compulsorily insured patients on the list, and a lower tariff for those exceeding this number. The fee consists of several elements: net income, pension contributions and practice costs. Tariffs are negotiated between the Association of General Practitioners and the Association of Sickness Funds and must be approved by the Ministry.

For tariffs for privately insured patients there is an analogous procedure with the coordinating office of insurance companies. Privately insured patients pay their general practitioner a fee-for-service, which may be reimbursed by their insurance company if these services are included in the package, and taking account of possible deductibles. Medical specialists receive fees, specified per item of care, from publicly as well as privately insured patients. Fees of general practitioners and specialists for the privately insured are higher than for those insured under the Sickness Funds. Hospital budgets are fixed annually. Tariffs are negotiated with financers and finally approved by the Central Agency of Health Care Tariffs. Wages for non-medical staff are the result of negotiations between labour unions and health care employers Pharmacists in extramural care receive a fee per prescription. This dispensing fee is negotiated between insurers and pharmacists and approved by the Central Agency of Health Care Tariffs.

3.6 *Policy developments in health care*

In the eighties the Dutch government decided to reform the health care system. The Dekker committee pinpointed five major problems in the system: a fragmented funding structure, the lack of solidarity in private health insurance, the lack of incentives for efficiency, the detailed government regulations and the increasing costs. With these shortcomings in mind the committee proposed a new basic health insurance package. This package includes more financial incentives for insurers, providers and consumers. At the heart of the reforms is the introduction of a basic health insurance package for all residents, covering the bulk of essential health and social services. This will account for approximately 90% of all current medical and social services, namely: general practitioner services, prescribed drugs, medical/ nursing aids and appliances, paramedical services, preventive care, obstetric and maternity services, nursing, treatment and care for the elderly and the mentally and physically handicapped, rehabilitation, medical and surgical treatment and associated short-term hospital stay, psychosocial care, dental care and transportation services.

Apart from the compulsory basic insurance, the insured person may opt for voluntary supplementary insurance covering provisions such as cosmetic surgery.

In the future system, the present sickness funds and private insurers will act as general health insurers. Patients will be free to choose their insurer. Insurers will be obliged to accept all applicants irrespective of risk and/or health status, and will not be allowed to differentiate premiums according to risk.

The premium to be paid is split into two parts. Citizens will pay a large proportion of the costs of health care (approximately 80%) as a percentage of their taxable income. This part, levied together with regular taxes by the tax department, will be deposited in a central fund. In addition, individuals will pay a flat rate premium directly to the insurer. The fixed premiums may vary, according to the coverage and the administrative efficiency of the insurer, but the insurers may not differentiate according to the perceived risk of a certain category of insured. They will receive fixed annual budgets from the central fund, related to the risk characteristics of their clients (age, sex, chronic disease, region). The insurers will enjoy more freedom of negotiation. The legal obligation to enter into contract with all potential providers of care will be abolished. This will clear the way for insurers to select the most efficient providers of care and to determine the best price-product ratio in order to reduce costs and flat premiums.

The new system will also contain incentives for consumers. Since 1-1-1992 all insurers haven been allowed to offer lower nominal premiums coupled to co-payment by the insured, who for example can accept responsibility for the first 500 or 1000 guilders of claims annually, in exchange for premium reduction.

The new health care system entails a shift of responsibilities from the government to other parties. The central government will no longer be responsible for setting charges and planning health care provisions. Government involvement will still be required in the following areas: the level of income-related premiums, type, content and volume of the basic health insurance package and the guidelines applying to the capitation payment system for insurers. On the other hand insurers, providers of care and consumers will assume greater responsibility for an accessible, affordable and good health care. These new relationships require strengthening of the position of the health care consumer. Financial support is given to consumers' and patients' organisations to develop their expertise. The Federation of Patients Organisations is officially represented in the Health Insurance Council and other advisory bodies. Legislation protecting patients' rights has been submitted to Parliament.

The Dutch government remains responsible for the quality of health care and is developing new legislation to ensure that quality systems are introduced in the health care sector. However, the concrete development and functioning of quality systems belong to the responsibilities of insurers, care providers and professionals. The government has opted for a step-by-step approach to modernising the health care system. The Exceptional Medical Expenses Act (AWBZ) should serve as a vehicle for the introduction of the basic health insurance package. Almost all medical services from the sickness funds and private insurance schemes will be incorporated in this package. The scope of the AWBZ was already expanded in 1989 and 1992. Capitation grants will gradually replace the present fee-for-service system.

Every step in this transformation process requires extensive political debate and consultation with all parties involved. Changes in law require extensive legislative procedures. This makes it difficult to predict a precise timetable. It is even difficult to predict the outcome of the proposed restructuring process. Changes in the political environment may cause changes in emphasis. The new cabinet, installed after the 1994 election, has announced it will strengthen the role of the general practitioner as "gatekeeper", abolish fee-for-service payments for specialists, equalize the position of sickness funds and private insurers, restrict the AWBZ package to uninsurable risks and care for the elderly, restrict the package of the compulsory insurance by removing dental care for adults, physiotherapy and other paramedical care and set limits for available drugs. Drugs and therapeutic appliances will return from the AWBZ to the normal insurance scheme. General deductibles of 200 guilders will be introduced, but co-payments are intended to be abolished. With these measures the new cabinet expects to limit the annual growth of health care expenditure to 1.3%.

3.7 *Organisation of health care*

3.7.1 *General characteristics*

Health care in the Netherlands is mainly supplied by private non-profit institutions and independent professionals. The health care system is often described as consisting of four so-called echelons.

- *The basic echelon* offers an open supply of collective prevention services: immunisation, school health care, industrial health care, health education. Municipalities fulfil the most important role with regard to collective prevention.
- *The first echelon* refers to the direct accessible care provided by general practitioners, dentists, pharmacists, physiotherapists, home care by the "Cross" and Home Help Organisations, midwives, speech therapists and others.
- *The second echelon*, only accessible after referral by the general practitioner, consists of extramural, independent specialists, out-patient departments and acute hospital care.
- *The third echelon*, also accessible after referral only, concerns long-term care in psychiatric hospitals, convalescence centres and nursing homes.

The general rule is that patients first visit their general practitioner. This procedure is mandatory under the sickness fund scheme, except in the case of emergency. Most private insurance companies also stipulate that patients should first consult the general practitioner. The general practitioner thus functions as the "gatekeeper" of the health care system. He can refer patients to independent specialists, out-patient departments, or to hospitals for admission.

General practitioners are informed by specialists of diagnosis and treatment so that they can take over the treatment when the patient is referred back. Patients who no longer need specialist care in the short stay hospitals, can be referred to nursing homes, convalescence centres or psychiatric hospitals. The general practitioner can also mobilize home care by the "Cross" organisations or refer to other professionals like physiotherapists.

3.7.2 *Intramural care*

Almost all hospitals (88%) and other services are private institutions, working on a non-profit base. The hospital system comprises general, categorial (single specialty) and university (teaching) hospitals. They all have out-patient departments, which form an integral part of the hospital system. Moreover psychiatric hospitals, institutes for the mentally deficient and nursing homes are counted under intramural care. In the past 15 years many hospitals have had to combine forces, resulting in a reduction in the number of beds. This has been compensated by promoting short-stay facilities and day care, and by on the one hand providing more diagnostic facilities to general practitioners while on the other reinforcing extramural care.

Most medical specialists work in hospitals. Two-thirds of them are free entrepreneurs, often working in partnerships. They have contracts with hospitals for the use of hospital facilities and employ their own staff.
In the Netherlands a distinction is made between intramural care and semi-mural care. Because this distinction is not known in other countries semi-mural care is discussed under intramural care.

The sector semi-mural care brings together different types of care for patients for whom complete hospitalization is not necessary or desirable and for whom normal out-patient services are insufficient. Patients are treated mainly during the daytime (except maternity clinics). Most of the services in this sector have medical and/or paramedical characteristics: maternity clinics, nurseries for toddlers under medical supervision, centres for convalescence day treatment, day centres for the disabled, abortion clinics and institutes for oncological and radiotherapeutical day treatment.

Private (for profit) clinics are also classified in this category, because they provide only day care treatment in plastic surgery, ophthalmology, dermatology, flebology and orthopaedics. In the case of the institutes for sensorily disabled, treatment and nursing is combined with education and professional training. In family replacement homes and regional institutes for supervised residence, psycho-therapy and social guidance is emphasized in combination with supervised residence. These institutes offer transitional care for discharged psychiatric patients. They also function as homes for lighter cases of mental deficiency with supporting care from an intramural setting.

3.7.3 Extramural care

Since the seventies the government has tried to advance cohesion in extramural care by stimulating teamwork. This policy has been partially successful. In 1995 there were 150 health centres, in which on average three to four general practitioners, a similar number of district nurses, one or two social workers and physiotherapists work together with supportive staff in shared premises.

More recent policy aims have resulted in a large number of substitution experiments in home care for the elderly, for terminally ill and early discharged patients.

3.7.3.1 Medical care

A typical Dutch general practitioner (GP) is independent, owns his own premises and is assisted by a receptionist or practice assistant (See literature no. 6). He serves an average population of 2,165 inhabitants (1995). For many diagnostic procedures general practitioners rely on external facilities. A diminishing proportion of general practitioners, now 11%, usually in rural areas, have a pharmacy of their own. A general practitioner is responsible for round the clock availability of service, seven days a week. This is usually achieved on a rota basis in local tenancy groups with other general practitioners in the area. House calls belong to the normal tasks. Although general practitioners are not involved in hospital treatment, they do visit hospitalised patients, but not as a rule.

Most GPs (54%) work alone, 31% work on a partnership basis and 16% work in a group practice. The practices of well over 8% of GPs are part of a health centre, which is mostly run by a private foundation or association and encouraged by government subsidies.

Independent specialists, working in their own premises, are especially found among ophthalmologists, dermatologists, allergologists, psychiatrists and orthodontists. Other specialists only work in hospitals and provide ambulatory care in the outpatient departments. Also specialists of the categories, mentioned above, can have their working place in hospitals and their outpatient departments.

3.7.3.2 *Dental care*

Most dentists in the Netherlands work in their own premises. They serve an average population of about 2100 inhabitants (1995). Others find employment in intramural care, Municipal Health Services (youth dental health), army, university, government, and health insurance funds.

The dentist in general practice is entitled to practice dentistry to its fully extent. His scope is not limited to "hard tissue" (teeth), but also concerns "soft tissue". Important tasks are the early detection of teeth defects, parodontal defects, defects of the mucous membrane and defects in the relation jaw muscles and joint. Like the general practitioner the dentist plays the role of "gatekeeper" in health care. The vast majority of the Dutch population visits his dentist regularly for preventive examination. Therefore, primary and secondary prevention are important characteristics of dental care. Main tasks of the dentist are:

- diagnostics;
- prevention;
- restorative care;
- prosthetic care;
- orthodontic care;
- surgical care.

3.7.3.3 *Pharmacists*

The qualified pharmacist is entitled to:

- the preparation of drugs and delivery, directly or after receipt;
- control and examination of drugs;
- surveillance of drugs use by patients (medication surveillance);
- consultation of physicians regarding pharmacotherapy;
- information about drugs for physicians;
- information about drugs for patients.

The vast majority of pharmacists work in the officinal pharmacy as the established pharmacist or as second pharmacist. Another part is employed as hospital pharmacist in intramural health care. Other fields of activity are industry and university.

The officinal pharmacist (established and second) serves an average population of 7256 inhabitants (1993).

3.7.3.4 Midwifery

Primary care obstetrics is mainly in the hands of midwives. About 30% of births take place at home. In the Dutch country profile midwifery is described distinctly, because midwifery is considered a medical profession in the Netherlands and therefore midwifery has a place in health care different from other countries. In the Netherlands midwives can be consulted without referral. They have an autonomous competence for judgement and decision (referral included) and the complete responsibility for antenatal, natal and postnatal care in low and medium-risk obstetrics, including the final inspection six weeks post partum. Furthermore, extramural midwives render services to women who had their child in an intramural institution (hospital, maternity clinic) and went home soon after the delivery. Midwives play an important advisory role in the field of family planning.

The vast majority of midwives (85%) is active in extramural care from own practices or practices shared with other midwives. A small group (15%) is employed by hospitals or is in a partnership with gynaecologists.

3.7.3.5 Paramedical care

Paramedical professions in the Netherlands are: physiotherapist, ergotherapist, speech therapist, dietician, therapist training method Cesar, therapist training method Mensendieck, dental hygienist and podotherapist.

After referral by a practising physician, the physiotherapist applies one or more of the following therapies: movement therapy, massage therapy and physical therapy in a strict sense i.e. the application of physical stimuli, electrotherapy, ultra-sound therapy, thermotherapy, hydrotherapy, balneotherapy and electrodiagnostics, with the exclusion of the application of ionising beams.

Most physiotherapists (70%) are active in extramural health care. They normally work in independent practices with one or more physiotherapists. The other part is employed in intramural institutions. A small group is active in the field of sports, occupational health, special schools and municipal health services.

After referral by a practising physician, the ergotherapist observes impediments in daily activities and labour, trains patients in coping with these impediments, whether or not with application of expedients, and advises patients with regard to living and working conditions and provisions needed.
Ergotherapists are employed in both extramural and intramural care, but predominantly in intramural institutions.

The speech therapist examines speech defects under the responsibility of a practising physician or dentist and improves speech abilities of patients by relief of deficiencies of breath regulation.

Speech therapists are active in the field of health care, both extramural and intramural, but also in other sectors. In extramural care they normally work in their own practices. In intramural care they are employed by hospitals, nursing homes, psychiatric institutions etc. In the education sector, speech therapists are active in primary and special education.

The dietician composes diets for medical purposes adjusted to patients under the responsibility of a physician or dentist and advises patients with regard to their diet.

Dieticians have a wide range of employment possibilities. They have independent practices in extramural care or may be employed by "Cross"-organisations. In preventive health care they may be employed in the field of health education and information. About 30% is working in extramural care, but 45%, however, is employed in intramural care (hospitals, nursing homes etc.). Others are employed in education, industry, research and government.

The therapist training method Cesar aims at the realisation of a motorial learning process, corresponding to diagnosis, the therapeutical goal, agreed with physician and patient, and the individual motorial capacities of the patient.

Cesar-therapists can be active in different fields of health care. The vast majority is self-employed in own practices. Furthermore, there are employment possibilities in intramural care (hospital rehabilitation hospital or nursing home), but also in preventive health care and education.

The therapist training method Mensendieck aims, after referral by a practising physician, at the realisation of self-analysis and correction of patient's attitude and movement in order to abate and prevent complaints regarding the motorial apparatus. Self-responsibility plays an important role in this method.

Mensendieck-therapists can be active in different fields of health care. The vast majority is self-employed in their own practices. Furthermore, there are employment possibilities in intramural care (hospital, rehabilitation hospital or nursing home), but also in preventive health care and education.

The dental hygienist examines teeth under the responsibility of a practising dentist and reports about dental conditions and surrounding tissues, cleans teeth, applies preserving and preventing means at teeth and surrounding tissues and provides patients with information regarding dental hygiene.

The majority of dental hygienists (80%) is employed in extramural care. Others are employed in intramural care or in professional training. Most dental hygienists are employed by dentists. A few are working in independent practices, treating patients after written referral by dentists or dental specialists.

After referral by a practising physician, the podotherapist applies corrective and protective therapies concerning foot functions, treats external defects of the skin of the foot and prevents and treats nail defects.

Podotherapists mostly work in extramural care (85%) in independent practices. Others (13%) are active in both extramural and intramural care and a few (2%) are employed in intramural care only.

3.7.3.6 Home nursing and home care 1)

Dutch community nursing care and home help services are organised on two main levels:

National level: National Association for Home Care
Regional level: 38 Regional Cross Organisations
Regional level: 85 Home help organisations
Regional level: 31 Home care organisations

The National Association for Home Care is an umbrella organisation for community nursing and home help services and has four duties:

- policy making on the national level;
- promotion of the interests of its members, i.e. the regional organisations;
- engaging in collective bargaining with government and insurance companies;
- provision of services to the Regional Cross Associations, home care and the home help organisations.

In 1990 the two umbrella organisations for community nursing and home help services were merged into the National Association for Home Care. At this moment this integration is also taking place at the regional level. It is expected that this integration will result in more efficiency in home care and will help avoid unnecessary overlap between home nursing and home help services. In the middle of 1993, 31 home care organisations had already been integrated, providing both community nursing and home help services. The 38 regional cross associations provide community nursing only and the 85 home help organisations provide home help services only.

Community nurses are employed by the Regional Cross Associations or by the integrated Home care organisations. The regional cross associations consist of a number of so-called basic units. A basic unit has a chief nursing officer (head nurse), about ten community nurses, and two or three auxiliary nurses work in a team. A basic unit is assigned to a defined geographical area (about 35000 inhabitants). Within this team each individual nurse, or a sub-team of a few nurses and an auxiliary nurse, is assigned to a specific sub-area. Most of the home care organisations have integrated teams in which community nurses and auxiliary nurses and qualified home helps work together. In addition there are separate teams of unqualified home helps, who mainly perform household tasks.

Regional cross associations and home care organisations can be reached 24- hours-a day and care can be provided in the evenings, nights and weekends if necessary. Patients are entitled to a maximum amount of nursing care at home: 2.5 hours a day or three visits a day, for an unlimited period of time.

Patients, who need more intensive home nursing for a limited period of time, mostly terminal patients or patients waiting for admission to a nursing home, can make an appeal to additional home care. This additional home care is provided by private organisations or by foundations related to the regional cross associations.

Because the regional cross associations and the home care organisations are the main providers of home nursing and also because there is no information about the number of private organisations for (intensive) home care, this description of home nursing in the Netherlands focus mainly on the Cross Associations and integrated home care organisations.

Patients can contact the cross associations or home care organisations themselves because no referral is needed. Traditionally, the assessment is carried out by a community nurse (first level nurse), who is also going to provide the nursing care or who delegates the care to a second level nurse. In the regional cross organisations this is still the case. However, most home care organisations, delivering home nursing as well as home help services, intend to combine the assessment of patient's need for help and for nursing care.

Community nurses (first level nurses) are qualified to perform all of the following tasks:

- assessment of the need of care;
- hygienic and other personal care (e.g. bathing, help with lavatory, help with activities of daily living);
- routine technical nursing procedures (such as injections, dressings, stoma care, bladder wash out);
- more complicated technical nursing (e.g. epidermal anaesthesia, handling respirator, and catheterization);

- patient education;
- psychosocial activities;
- encouraging help e.g. from family members, neighbours, friends etc.;
- evaluation of care.

Auxiliary nurses (second level) are also qualified to perform most of the tasks mentioned above, except the assessment of the need of care, more complicated technical nursing procedures and the evaluation of care. In addition, auxiliaries more often provide hygiene care and usually do not provide psychosocial support.

Home helps are employed by the home help organisations or by the integrated home care organisations. Most of the home care organisations have integrated teams in which community nurses and auxiliary community nurses and qualified home helps work together. In addition they have separate teams of unqualified home helps, who only carry out household tasks. Traditionally in most home help organisations (qualified) home helps do not work in teams, they work as soloists.

In most regions of the Netherlands there is only one home help or home care organisation. Consequently, people formally do not have a choice when they need home help services.

No formal referral is needed, so potential clients can contact the home help services directly. Traditionally, the assessment of needs is made by a home help organiser, mostly someone with a training in social work, who is not involved in direct patient care. Most integrated home care organisations have chosen a special assessment team consisting of a few persons with a nursing background and a few persons with experience in assessing needs for home help services (mostly social workers).

After the assessment the care is allocated by the home help organiser. Because there are waiting lists the most desirable amount of care can not always be provided and dependent on the urgency of the needs, most clients have to wait a number of weeks or even months before they actually receive the assessed care. Reassessment is made by the home help organiser at least twice a year. The actual home help is provided by different categories of home helps: qualified home helps, unqualified home helps and "alpha-helps", the latter being home helps for a maximum of twelve hours a week, which is the limit below which they do not have to pay social security contributions.

3.7.3.7 Maternity home care

A particular aspect of home care is maternity home care. Maternity centres provide qualified personnel for the assistance of midwives or general practitioners during the confinement and for the care for mother and child during a week after the delivery especially with regard to home deliveries or maternity care at home after intramural confinement. These maternity centres function under the auspices of the National Association for Home Care.

3.7.3.8 *Extramural mental health care services*

The most important categories of mental health care institutions are:

- Regional institutions for ambulatory mental health care (RIAGG);
- Consultation Bureaus for Alcohol and Drugs Addicts;
- Out-patient departments of psychiatric and general hospitals;
- Independent psychiatrists.

a. *Regional institutions for mental health care (RIAGG)*

There are 58 regions, from 150.000 to 300.000 inhabitants, in which extramural mental health care is provided by a regional institution for ambulatory mental health care (RIAGG). Within this institution distinct teams are functioning for youth, adults, the elderly and psychotherapy. Around the clock service is offered during 7 days a week. Immediate access is possible (no referral is needed), but patients also are referred to the RIAGG by general practitioners, visiting nurses, social welfare, school health, home help services etc.

The work of the RIAGG can be divided into three main tasks: treatment, prevention and services. Treatment comprises intake and examination, followed by referral, mediation, consultancy or treatment. Treatment can be given to persons of all age categories with psychiatric and psychosocial problems. During the treatment attention is paid to psychological, biological and social aspects of complaints.

The aim of prevention is to further, that people learn to sort out their life and social problems themselves. Assistance should be supplied by people in their immediate environment. Preventive projects are directed to change the social systems in which people live. An example of a preventive project is the prevention of psychiatric hospital admission.

RIAGG services can be divided into internal and external services. Internal services comprise supervision, intervision, advising and consultation. External services are mainly consultation activities, supporting extramural health care workers (general practitioners, school health, home nursing) in their responsibility for people with psychosocial complaints.

The RIAGG has an obligatory connection with the Consultation Bureau's for alcohol and drugs.

b. *Consultation Bureau's for alcohol and drugs*
There are 17 Consultation Bureau's for alcohol and drug addicts with all together 64 establishments.

The treatment by these institutions is directed to the physical aspects of alcohol and drug abuse, but also to the underlying psychological problems, which are part of addicts' behaviour and social background problems. Specialist teams are operating for alcohol addicts and drug addicts.

Direct access is possible, but many people are referred by social welfare institutions, other mental health care institutions, municipal health services and the like. Treatment is without financial consequences for the patient. The financing of these institutions is the responsibility of the Ministry of Health, Welfare and Sports and the Ministry of Justice.

c. *Out-patient departments of psychiatric and general hospitals*
Outpatient departments of psychiatric and general hospitals are therapeutical provisions for patients with psychic and psychiatric problems who do not need intensive or specialist treatment. One category of patients is those who are discharged from intramural care, the other is referred to by e.g. general practitioners. Though all outpatient departments are connected with a hospital, not all are part of the hospital complex. Sometimes they have been established in "outstations", located elsewhere.

d. *Independent psychiatrists*
About 1100 psychiatrists are operating independently and yet are contracted by health insurance funds. Many of them combine this independent practice with a job in a hospital, RIAGG, or other institution, so that in fact about 300 FTE's are active. Patients, adults as well as children, normally are referred by general practitioners. After examination the psychiatrist advises the general practitioner, refers to another institution or continues treatment.

Government policy is directed to co-operation agreements of these independent psychiatrists with RIAGG.

3.7.3.9 Ambulance services and patient transport
The fields of activity of the "Centrale Posten Ambulancevervoer" (CPA's) (Central Post for Ambulance Services) is determined by the provinces who draft a plan with respect to the number of ambulances and in the distribution.

Local authorities are obliged to work together in the organisation of the CPA's. These posts not only receive emergency calls, but requests for regular ambulance transport pass through these offices. Transport and transporters are delegated and directed from these CPA's. These transporters may be private companies, Municipal Health Services or hospitals.

Ambulances are exclusively used for recumbent transport. Furthermore, there is also the so-called transport of patients in a sitting position, for which taxis can be used, or in the case of handicapped persons, wheelchair buses. Health insurance funds pay for this if transport is medically necessary, and the patient has paid the yearly contribution of Dfl. 139.50 (1995). In some cases, compensation may be paid to patients using their own private car.

In most cases persons who are privately insured must pay a certain percentage constituting their "own risk" for all provisions, including patient transport.

3.7.3.10 Medical laboratories

For their support regarding diagnostic tests, general practitioners can make use of a variety of institutions. Hospital facilities (e.g. radiation, clinical chemistry) are at their disposal and sometimes hospitals compiled their diagnostic capacity in the so-called "diagnostic centre" of the hospital. Diagnostic centres have also been established outside hospital. Moreover, there are (juridical) independent medical laboratories and medical laboratories, which are incorporated in hospital organisations and which often are connected with a thrombosis service.

Blood samples can be taken at the laboratory, but also at geographically dispersed locations and at the patients' home, if the necessity is indicated by the general practitioner.

Services that can be rendered to the general practitioner are:

- clinical chemical tests;
- haematological tests;
- bacteriological and serological tests;
- examination of urine, faeces, stomach content;
- ECG (including judgement of the results).

3.8 *Preventive health care*

Many government and non-government organisations play a role in the field of prevention and health protection. Traditionally health protection is the role of central government (e.g. monitoring of food, drinking water, and environmental protection), but tasks also have been delegated to lower authorities. Local authorities and their Municipal Health Services (GGD's) are charged by law with collective prevention, but private organisations, are also active. The Municipal Health Services are responsible for school health (4–19 years), youth dental hygiene, prevention of

TBC, sexually transmitted diseases and AIDS, environmental hygiene and psycho-hygiene (in co-operation with RIAGG's), preventive programs, health education and information and epidemiology.

The national immunisation program is carried out by the "cross" organisations under supervision of the National Institute of Public Health and the Environment. The "cross" organisations also provide preventive care for children (0-4 years), including PKU/CHT screening and early detection of developmental disorders.

Voluntary organisations are active in many fields e.g. the promotion of screening for breast and cervical cancer, the prevention of addiction (drugs, alcohol, tobacco and gambling) and mental problems like depression and suicide. General practitioners take cervical smears in the prevention program of cervical cancer and they also give flu vaccination for seniors.

Occupational health care is mainly provided by independent services on behalf of civil service, business, trade and industry.

3.9 *Medical goods*

Medical goods include two categories: the category of pharmaceuticals and the category of therapeutic appliances.

3.9.1 *Pharmaceuticals*

Pharmaceuticals in the Netherlands include pharmaceuticals in a strict sense as well as wound dressings and bandages.

Pharmaceuticals in a strict sense are divided in pharmaceuticals on prescription (of a medical profession), pharmaceuticals obligatory supplied by a pharmacist (or a dispensing physician) and over the counter medicines. This last category can be freely sold in a drugstore or in any other shop. Wound dressings and bandages can be freely sold by any retailer.

To control the expenditure on pharmaceuticals the government fixed the prices. This means that the average in a group of equal therapeutic value determines the price. If more expensive drugs are chosen the patient must pay the difference.

3.9.2 *Therapeutic appliances*

Therapeutic appliances in the Netherlands contain all kind of devices for performing a certain physical function. These devices range from glasses to artificial legs and wheel chairs. Most therapeutic appliances are especially made to order or adapted to the patient by specialised professionals or specialised companies.

3.10 *Other services*

Other services consist of activities that in general are not being defined as health care in a strict sense, but of activities of which the costs are adopted in the national health accounts of many countries.

Other services consist of the administrative expenditures in the health care sector (an integral part of the Dutch health accounts), and the expenditures on Research & Development and the expenditures on Training & Education in health care. These last two subjects are no part of the Dutch health accounts.

Note

[1] This paragraph is derived from literature no. 26.

4. Country profile: Denmark

4.1 Introduction

The exchange of information in the network of experts facilitated the production of the "country profiles", which are meant to provide:

- a quick introduction to the organisation and administration of the health care systems of the participating countries;
- an exploration of the boundaries of the health care systems;
- a preliminary determination of place and functions of health care;
- an overview of the main policy developments;
- a contribution to transparency, a necessary condition for international comparison.

The country profiles contain information on health care administration, financing, policy developments and the organisation of health care. This information was brought together in the two phases of the project "international comparison of health care data".

In the first phase (1994–1995) the boundaries of the national health care systems were explored. Also general characteristics of health care administration, financing, policy developments and health care organisation were described.

Detailed quantative data became available on intramural health care. The expression "ïntramural health care" proved to be a typically Dutch one. Intramural health care is by and large equal to in-patient health care or stationary care. The description used (see Annex 2.4) is health care for patients formally admitted for a period of more than 24 hours and/or institutionalised treatment for a substantial part of the day (or night).

In the second phase of the project (1996–1997) more detailed data were collected on extramural care, preventive health care, medical goods and other services. Also attention was paid to an update of the determination of the boundaries of national health care systems.

Also the expression "extramural health care" proved to be a typically Dutch one. Extramural health care is described as health care provided on a non-residential basis by medical and paramedical professionals or by specialised organisations in home care or home nursing (for a complete description see Annex 2.4).

At the start of the project the intention was to provide country profiles for all the sectors of care described in this report. This goal was not reached. Especially

information on the topic of "other services" is lacking. To a lesser extent the same holds true for the topic of "medical goods".

The country profile of Denmark was edited by Ms. M. Kruse of Denmark.

4.2 *Aspects of general administration of health care*

In Denmark health care is mainly the responsibility of the national, regional and local authorities. At national level the Ministry of Health is the main authority and is responsible for legislation on health care, personnel, hospitals and pharmacies, pharmaceutical products, nutrition, vaccination, maternity and child care, patient rights etc. The Ministry controls the health care system mainly by issuing general rules and guidelines. Its main advisor is the National Board of Health; this agency also fulfils advisory tasks for local authorities and health professionals. In addition to advisory tasks the National Board carries out the administration of health services, supervisory functions with regard to health professionals and is charged with regulation and planning of the education of health professionals. The only executive task of the Ministry of Health with regard to health care is the operation and management of the National University Hospital in Copenhagen, which serves as a model for regional hospitals. Due to the organisational reform of the Copenhagen area, mentioned later, this task will end at the beginning of 1995, when this hospital will function as "Capital Hospital".

The 16 counties in Denmark play the most important role in the field of health care. They are responsible for hospital care and primary curative care as well as for health promotion activities. At local level, the 275 municipalities are responsible for the care for the elderly, including both home nursing services and nursing homes, and a number of preventive programmes including public health nurses, school health and child dental services.

4.3 *Financing of health care*

As most health care services are free of charge, the major part of health care spending, about 85%, is public expenditure, borne by general taxation (state, county, municipality). The counties play the most important role in financing health care. Public spending on hospitals as wel as the Health Care Reimbursement Scheme are financed by the counties and account for 65% of total county spending.

In order to distribute the burden of hospital and other costs more equally, "block grants" are paid by the national government to the counties, based on differences in income levels of the inhabitants and demographic characteristics.
These grants represent about 25% of the health care spending by counties. Private expenditure amounts to about 15% of total health care expenditure. Co-payments and over the counter expenses constitute 92% of these private expenditures, private insurance the remaining 8%.

4.4 *Insurance structure*

Most health care services are provided by counties and municipalities as a public service free of charge. All hospital services (in-patient and out-patient) and municipal health care services are free at the point of use, as are curative services by general practitioners and specialists under the Health Care Reimbursement Scheme.

Private health insurance is mainly supplied by one non-profit insurance company called "Danmark". About 26% of the population is covered by "Danmark".

4.4.1 *Sickness fund benefits*

Under the Health Care Reimbursement Scheme citizens can choose between two types of arrangements, group 1 and group 2. The majority of the population (in 1991 96.4%) chose group 1.

Group 1 patients are registered with one specific general practitioner, which they may consult free of charge. If group 1 patients need to see a practising specialist, a referral by their general practitioner (GP) is necessary to get specialist treatment free of charge. Group 2 patients are free to visit any GP or practising specialist without previous referral. Group 2 patients receive reimbursement equivalent to the reimbursement given to group 1, but in this case doctors are free to charge extra. Also co-payments for medication and dental services are higher for group 2 patients.

If a GP has 1325 patients, he may close his list. If a GP has 2096 adult group 1 patients, his list is closed until the number is less than 1988.

The private insurer "Danmark" offers three different degrees of protection. Two are meant as a supplement to group 1 in the Health Care Reimbursement Scheme. The other is a supplement to group 2 in the Health Care Reimbursement Scheme. Most of the reimbursements by "Danmark" are for medication and dental care, not fully covered by the Health Care Reimbursement Scheme.

4.4.2 *Cost sharing*

Co-payments exist for some services under the Health Care Reimbursement Scheme, particularly for medication (outside the hospital), dental services, physiotherapy etc.

The Health Care Reimbursement Scheme partly reimburses expenditure on medication prescribed by physicians or dentists if included in two specific lists published by the Ministry of Health. For drugs included in the lists the reimbursement is 75% and 50% respectively. The scheme also partly reimburses specific types of dental care, while other types of dental care are paid for entirely by the patients.

4.5 *Fee and salary structure*

Doctors and other hospital staff are salaried employees. The salaries are negotiated centrally by the County Councils Association and the trade unions. Hospital specialists may be allowed to do private outpatient care for up to three hours a week at hospitals; these specialists then pay rent for hospital facilities. Their services are usually paid for by the Health Care Reimbursement Scheme. Costs of private hospitals are paid at the same rate as public hospitals. Extra bills must be paid by the patients themselves. Office-based general practitioners and specialists run a private practice. The main part of their income comes from the Health Care Reimbursement Scheme. General practitioners are paid according to a combined capitation/ fee-for-service scheme.

Office-based specialists are paid on a pure fee-for-service basis. Fees are negotiated between providers, professional organisations and the Association of County Councils. The contracts specify prices for all services covered and imply that fees and capitation are paid by the counties in full or in part. In the latter case the remainder must be paid by the patients directly. No extra billing is allowed for services covered by the contracts.

With regard to pharmacists the Ministry of Health negotiates their total gross profit and a corresponding mark-up scale with the pharmacists association.

Staff in the municipal health care services (home nurses, public health nurses, school health services and child dental care) are salaried employees. Salaries are negotiated centrally by trade unions and the Association of Municipalities.

4.6 *Policy developments in health care*

Cost containment policy is considered to have been successful in Denmark. One basic reason for this is the financing of health care by counties and municipalities, which have been under economic restraint by the national government. In the last decade many activities have also been initiated to improve the efficiency of health care services by developing information systems, modernising hospital administration and management and organising work and training programmes more effectively. Extra attention has been paid to general practitioners. Hospital facilities – such as consultancy and the use of laboratories – have been put at their disposal.

Furthermore municipal home nursing services offer a twenty-four hour service so that referral to hospital can be prevented and patients can stay at home.

In the near future further improvements are expected as consequences of the introduction of a competition element, more free choice for patients and market orientation. Concrete plans have been developed to reduce waiting lists, not only on the part of the hospital, but also on the part of the municipal home nursing service. Since 1993 Counties are allowed to charge municipalities for the costs of patients having to wait in hospital after treatment for the municipal home nursing service to take over.

From January 1995 the hospitals of Copenhagen and Frederiksberg and the State University Hospital are joined in a company owned by the three parties together. This organisational reform, it is hoped, will pave the way for better resource utilisation in the Copenhagen area.

As part of the negotiations on the budget of 1995 Parliament has decided to introduce a new payment system for two specific operations, "slipped disc surgery" and "knee-alloplastic surgery". Patients on a waiting list for one of these treatments will be guaranteed treatment within three months from the time of referral by their general practitioner. If they cannot be treated in one of the wards of the home county within this time limit, the County is obliged to pay for treatment outside the County, either in another County hospital or in a private hospital/clinic. The prices of treatment are set at national level and the payment will be directed to the hospital treating the patient. Until now payments between County hospitals were payments between County-level budgets. This experiment came into effect in the spring of 1995. Other market-like incentives will be studied in the near future:

- development of a system of diagnosis related normal costs to facilitate comparisons of efficiency between hospitals and their departments and to support budgeting.
- improvement and expansion of data collection on output, costs etc., including registration of activities of general practitioners.
- investigation of the effects of contracting between Counties and hospitals, which already is taking place in some of the Counties.
- development of quality measures and improved information to the public to support the free choice in the framework of hospital reform.

4.7 *Organisation of health care*

4.7.1 *General characteristics*

Intramural care is operated mainly by regional and local authorities. Private hospitals are rare: in 1991 there were six, of which two can be characterized as proper acute hospitals and the others as specialised clinics for rheumatism (two), diabetes (one) and epilepsy (one). Extramural care is provided by self-employed professionals (general practitioners, practising specialists, dentists, physiotherapists, pharmacists) and public domain services (municipal home nursing services).

The general practitioner (GP) is the "gatekeeper" in the Danish health care system. Every patient must contact his or her GP. If the GP considers it necessary, the patient will be referred for further examination or treatment, either to a self-employed practising specialist or to a hospital. The GP may also call on the services of physiotherapists, health visitors, home nurses and the community social services. There are only few deviations from the this system:

- in the case of sudden serious injury or disease a patient may be treated at a hospital without any previous contact with the GP;
- referral is not necessary for eye specialists and ear, nose and throat specialists;
- in general referral is not necessary for "group 2" patients in the Health Care Reimbursement Scheme.

4.7.2 *Intramural care*

Almost all hospitals are owned and run by the counties. For hospital services that require larger catchment populations than one county an "inter-county market" has been established. From 1 January 1993 Danish citizens who need hospital treatment may choose from all public hospitals and a number of private clinics which co-operate with the public hospital services. This means that, after referral by his or her GP, the patient may choose the hospital without regard to geographical considerations. The county of residence will be obliged to pay for the treatment. Admission to highly specialised wards is granted only on medical grounds.

The hospitals cover the whole spectrum of physical and mental illness, providing diagnosis, treatment and care. They also provide diagnostic assistance to general practitioners on a considerable scale through laboratory services and imaging diagnostic services. The hospital services within a county consist of hospitals of different sizes and types. In general all major medical specialisms are offered by the hospital services of a given county. General hospitals with specialised departments constitute the largest group. Except for psychiatric hospitals, mono-specialised hospitals are almost non-existent. Nursing homes and institutions for the mentally handicapped are not considered to be part of health care services, but of the social welfare system at municipal level.

In the last decade hospitals have increasingly extended outpatient treatment in order to relieve the pressure on the in-patient facilities. Between 1980 and 1992 the total number of hospital beds decreased by 35%, from 41,500 to 27,000, and, counting only somatic beds, by 26%, from 32,500 to 24,000.

The number of admissions increased by 15% in the same period; this was accompanied by a rapid decline of the average length of stay, which is now under seven days (excluding psychiatry), and a corresponding expansion of outpatient services.

4.7.3 *Extramural care*

Extramural health care is a central and integral part of the Danish health care system. Extramural care is provided by self-employed professionals (general practitioners, practising specialists, dentists, physiotherapists, psychologists, chiropractors, chiropodists, pharmacists) and public domain services (municipal home nursing services and nursing homes).

Over the past decade much has been done to redistribute services from hospitals to the extramural health care sector.

4.7.3.1 Medical care

The pillar of the health care system is the so-called "family-doctor system". The general practitioner (GP) is the "gatekeeper" in the Danish health care system. Every patient must contact his or her GP in case of illness or injury. If the GP considers it necessary, the patient will be referred for further examination or treatment, either to a self-employed practising specialist or to a hospital. The GP may also call on the services of physiotherapists, health visitors, home nurses and the community social services.

There are only few deviations from this system: in the case of sudden serious injury or disease a patient may be treated at a hospital emergency ward without any previous contact with the GP;

Referral is not necessary for eye specialists and ear, nose and throat specialists; - in general referral is not necessary for "group 2" patients in the Health Care Reimbursement Scheme.

Everyone aged 16 or over may choose his or her own general practitioner. Families often keep the same family doctor for a number of years, which gives the doctor a thorough knowledge of the family's social and medical condition. In principle the general practitioner runs a private practice alone or in collaboration with other general practitioners.

Specialists examine and treat patients referred to them by general practitioners. There are about 800 full-time self-employed practising specialists in Denmark. A similar number have other positions, usually within the hospital services and have a private practice on a part-time basis.

Hospital specialists (hospital consultants) may be allowed to do private outpatient care for up to three hours a week at hospitals; these specialists then pay rent for hospital facilities. Their services are usually paid for by the Health Care Reimbursement Scheme.

Office-based general practitioners and specialists run a private practice. The main part of their income comes from the Health Care Reimbursement Scheme.

General practitioners are paid according to a combined capitation/fee-for -service scheme. Office-based specialists are paid on a pure fee-for-service basis.

4.7.3.2 *Dental care*

Most dentists have private practices and patients are free to choose. The Health Care Reimbursement Scheme also partly reimburses specific types of dental care, while other types of dental care are paid for entirely by the patients. Dental care for children and some elderly people is free of charge. The private insurance scheme 'Danmark' reimburses some of patient's expenditure on dentist's services.

4.7.3.3 *Pharmacists*

Pharmacists are independent entrepreneurs, but under considerable public control. The Ministry of Health determines the number and location of pharmacies and appoints new pharmacists.

The Ministry of Health negotiates their total gross profit and a corresponding mark-up scale with the pharmacists association.

4.7.3.4 *Paramedical care*

GPs can refer patients for treatment by physiotherapists and chiropractors, which are permitted to establish private practices. Physiotherapists may also be employed by municipalities, for instance in nursing homes. The Health Care Reimbursement Scheme only partly reimburses treatment by a private practising physiotherapist, psychologist, chiropodist or chiropractor.

4.7.3.5 *Home nursing and home care* [1)]

With the exception of acute hospital care, psychiatric institutions and general care (GP's), which are the county's responsibility, all remaining care for the elderly is organised by the municipality (Kommune). This implies that a broad range of facilities can be offered, while, according to priorities determined at community level, the emphasis can be on residential services, home care or other facilities. However, in general, absolute priority has been given to home care and sheltered housing. The Social Security Act of 1976 stresses the explicit obligation of the municipalities to organise home help services for the elderly. Nursing homes for elderly people are no longer built in Denmark. The building stop of nursing homes was introduced in the Social Security Act in 1988 in connection with a new act on housing for elderly people. In accordance with this act, from 1988 an increasing number of new sheltered dwellings for elderly people have been build. Several nursing home 'beds' were closed and replaced by sheltered housing. The sheltered housing is designed and produced in such a way, that the special needs of elderly and disabled people are taken into account. The elderly and disabled people are, in these settings, closely linked to staff and other service facilities.

In Denmark home nursing is provided by the municipality in the same department as home help services. Home nursing services are provided by home nurses and assistant nurses. The demand for home nursing care is generally initiated by health professionals.

The assessment procedures of home nursing needs can differ between the municipalities. Home nursing is granted on referral from a physician. Hospitals often use the services of a social counsellor for the estimation of the home care required and the contacts with the home care providers. In other cases there are fixed agreements, such as a nurse assessing home care needs on the same day or the day after discharge. In general, there is no formalised assessment: nurses assess the need for care and provide it themselves or have it provided by assistant nurses and/or home helps.

As already mentioned, home help and home nursing are organised within the community. Essential for the organisation of health care and social security in Denmark is the supply of a comprehensive and integrated set of services ranging from institutional care (nursing homes) to home help and from specially adapted housing facilities to concrete adaptations in existing dwellings. Since the building stop for nursing homes in 1988, there is an increased emphasis on home care facilities like home nursing and home help.

Home help, in its turn, belongs to an even wider range of services: neighbourhood work that includes services like gardening, snow clearance, meals-on-wheels and public transport for which modest co-payments are charged.

The help is to be granted and planned in close co-operation with the beneficiary and shall support him or her in preserving or regaining a physical and mental functional level. The provisions in the Social Security Act on home help are: home help of temporary or permanent character, home help for occasional relief, partial grant costs for help arranged by the beneficiary.
In the Social Security Act of 1976 the flowing home help activities have been described:

- housework such as cleaning, cooking, bed making, washing and ironing;
- assisting with going to the toilet, dressing, washing, bathing, hair combing and other aspects of personal hygiene;
- shopping and outdoor walks.

It is clear, that home help in Denmark involves substantially more, than just cleaning the house. Personal care such as dressing, washing, bathing re activities assigned to assistant nurses in most countries; while accompanying a disabled or frail person on outdoor walks and taking care of hopping is usually not included in home help activities in other countries that are ore strictly limited to cleaning activities.

4.7.3.6 Extramural mental health care services

The district psychiatry scheme, which is organised on county level, is a service for mentally ill people, who do not need to be admitted into psychiatric hospital. The district psychiatry scheme provides medication and medical attention when needed. Practising psychologists are free enterprises. Patients can attend a private psychologist without referral, and cost are not reimbursed. Only in the case of shock treatment following traffic accidents or other traumatic incidents, patients can be referred to treatment at a practising psychologist with partial reimbursement. These costs are held at county level. Practising psychiatrists are office-based specialists and as such observe the same conditions as other specialists mentioned under 'medical care'.

4.7.3.7 Extramural centres for alcohol and drugs addicts

A large number of private institutions are functioning in this area. These are to some degree supported financially by the state. On municipal level, also a few public institutions exist. These uphold primarily the function of hostels, however medical attention and treatment is offered as well.

4.7.3.8 Ambulance services and patient transport

The ambulance service is organised at county level. The service is entirely financed by the counties. Though the responsibility belongs to the counties, most counties have subcontracted this enterprise to the private organisation "Falck". Falck covers about 85 % of the population. The patient transport in counties or areas, not covered by Falck, is managed by the local fire brigade. All services are paid for from general taxation, and at no cost to the patient.

There is also a regulation governing the transport of seated patients. Wheelchair patients are compensated for the use of wheelchair buses. Subject to income (e.g. in the case of pensioners) some patients are eligible for compensation for transport by taxi. Transport in own cars can be reimbursed under certain conditions.

4.7.3.9 Medical laboratories

In most counties the laboratories are situated and run by hospitals. However in Copenhagen the general practitioners own a laboratory, to which they can refer patients for tests. All laboratory services are free for the patients.

4.8 *Preventive health care*

Denmark has several preventive health services, which are part of the established health care system and are free of charge.
Prenatal care and guidance can be obtained from the family doctor and from a midwife at a local midwifery centre and from hospitals. Several examinations are offered before and after delivery. During pregnancy prenatal diagnostic screening is offered to most women.

The municipal health authorities are notified of all births and offer the mother and child health care from a visiting public health nurse. All children are visited several times during their first year, depending on the need of the individual child or family. The main focus of the public health nurse is monitoring the child's health, advising and supporting the parents and providing information about supplementary health services. All children are entitled to preventive health examinations by a doctor. The first is scheduled for five weeks after birth.

All children (age under 18) are offered free immunisation by the family doctor against diphtheria, polio, tetanus, whooping cough, measles, mumps and German measles. Immunisation against German measles is also offered to women past the age of 12, as well as immunisation against the infectious disease caused by "haemophilus influenza, type B (HIB)" is offered to children younger than 6 years. A small number of children are now immunised against tuberculosis. The municipalities are responsible for the medical examination of all school children. In addition, all school children are examined in their first and last school year by a doctor employed by the municipality. The doctor and the school nurse participate in health education together with the teaching staff.
All children up to 18 years have access to free routine dental examinations and treatment. A preventive programme is carried out in day care institutions and schools. The dental care is provided by practising dentists or special services organised by the municipalities.

The occupational health services are separate from the ordinary health services. Their purpose is to prevent diseases and accidents at the workplace. Legislation sets certain standards for occupational safety and health facilities in factories and offices.

A wide range of other preventive measures have been established. Many of these were initiated by individual counties and municipalities and thus cover only the local area. National preventive measures include:

- sex education in all schools, including advice on contraception and sexually transmitted diseases.
- anonymous testing for human immunodeficiency virus (HIV) antibodies, free of charge.

A health promotion programme was presented to parliament in 1989. This programme defines the targets and initiatives of the national authorities. One basic idea of the programme is that a significant part of the health promotion tasks should be initiated locally, in close co-operation with people in the community and the local authorities and associations. The Minister for Health has set up an independent Council on Health Promotion Policy. An independent Council on Alcohol has been set up under this council.

Other national agencies for prevention and health promotion are:
- the National Board of Health;
- the Danish Council on Smoking;
- the Danish Veterinary and Food Administration;
- the Danish Institute for Clinical Epidemiology;
- the State Serum Institute;
- the Drugs Council.

4.9 *Medical goods*

Medical goods include two categories: the category of pharmaceuticals and the category of therapeutic appliances.

4.9.1 *Pharmaceuticals*

Pharmaceuticals, prices and profits

The wholesale profits are fixed through individual negotiations between each single manufacturer or importer and wholesaler and the profit level will be determined only by competition.

Pharmacy retail prices are calculated on a regressive scale set by the Ministry of Health. The retail prices consist of the pharmacy purchase price (the recommended price for the wholesalers' resale) plus a fixed amount and a percentage profit.

Reimbursement mechanisms

Reimbursement of the cost of medicinal products is administered by the county councils. At the pharmacy the patient only pays his share according to the reimbursement status of the product, and the pharmacy gets the reimbursement amount from the county.

Citizens may take out an insurance with the private insurance company "danmark" and thus obtain further reimbursement on presenting the bill from the pharmacy.

100% reimbursement is granted for insulin preparations. In all other cases decision concerning the reimbursement status of a given product depends on a concrete assessment along the following lines:

Generally a 49.8% reimbursement is granted for medicinal products which have a definite and valuable therapeutic effect, unless there is a risk of undesirable excess consumption. Generally a 74.7% reimbursement is granted for medicinal products which in addition to the above mentioned criteria are used for the treatment of well-defined and often life-threatening diseases; but only if the medicinal product in question may not be prescribed for less appropriate indications.

Medicinal products which may be bought without prescription may be added to the list of reimbursement of medicinal products. In such cases the reimbursement of 49.8% or 74.7%, however, is granted only to pensioners and patients suffering from chronic disease and only if a prescription has been issued for the medicinal product in question.

The Minister for Health may omit to grant reimbursement for a given medicinal product if the price of this product is not commensurate with its therapeutic value.

Reference price system
As mentioned above the reimbursement granted varies and may amount to 100%, 74.7% or 49.8% of the pharmacy retail price of a given product. If, however, several products contain the same active substance, reimbursement is granted in the form of *a fixed amount*. This is calculated as 100%, 74.7% or 49.8% of the average of the price of the two cheapest products in the group under consideration – the reference price. The fixed amount may not exceed 100%, 74.7% or 49.8% respectively of the retail price of a given product.

4.9.2 *Therapeutic appliances*
Purchase of many therapeutic appliances are partly reimbursed, if the patient is elderly or poor, and if the appliance is prescribed by a doctor, dentist, hearing therapist etc. Glasses and dental appliances are also partly reimbursed by the private insurance scheme 'Danmark'.

4.10 *Other services*
Other services consist of activities, that in general are not be defined as health care in a strict sense, but of activities, of which the costs are adopted in the national health accounts of many countries.

In the Danish health accounts official government expenditures in the administrative area are included, as are expenditures in the filed of health research performed in universities and the non-academic health education.

Note

1) This paragraph is derived from literature no. 63.

5. *Country profile: Germany*

5.1 *Introduction*

The exchange of information in the network of experts facilitated the production of the "country profiles", which are meant to provide

- a quick introduction to the organisation and administration of the health care systems of the participating countries;
- an exploration of the boundaries of the health care systems;
- a preliminary determination of place and functions of health care
- an overview of the main policy developments;
- a contribution to transparency, a necessary condition for international comparison.

The country profiles contain information on health care administration, financing, policy developments and the organisation of health care. This information was brought together in the two phases of the project "international comparison of health care data".

In the first phase (1994–1995) the boundaries of the national health care systems were explored. Also general characteristics of health care administration, financing, policy developments and health care organisation were described.

Detailed quantitative data became available on intramural health care. The expression "intramural health care" proved to be a typically Dutch one. Intramural health care is by and large equal to in-patient health care or stationary care. The description used (see Annex 2.4) is health care for patients formally admitted for a period of more than 24 hours and/or institutionalised treatment for a substantial part of the day (or night).

In the second phase of the project (1996–1997) more detailed data were collected on extramural care, preventive health care, medical goods and other services. Also attention was paid to an update of the determination of the boundaries of national health care systems.

Also the expression "extramural health care" proved to be a typically Dutch one. Extramural health care is described as health care provided on a non-residential basis by medical and paramedical professionals or by specialised organisations in home care or home nursing (for a complete description see Annex 2.4).

At the start of the project the intention was to provide country profiles for all the sectors of care described in this report. This goal was not reached. Especially

information on the topic of "other services" is lacking. To a lesser extent the same holds true for the topic of "medical goods".

The country profile of Germany was edited and completed by Dr. G. Brückner.

5.2 *Aspects of general administration of health care*

In the Constitution of the German Federal Republic some tasks in the field of public health are laid down. The principle of competing legislation is applied. This means, that the "Länder" have legislative competence in the absence of regulations at federal level. So considerable power has been delegated to the 16 Länder, especially with regard to hospital planning. In fact each level of government has distinct responsibilities:

- The federal government is responsible for drafting laws, for general policy and for jurisdiction over the health insurance system;
- The governments of the Länder are responsible for approving federal legislation, for the local supervision of sickness funds and physicians' associations, for managing the Länder-owned hospitals (including teaching hospitals), for hospital planning, for all investment in hospitals accredited by the Land plan and for regulating standards of medical education and the enrolment of medical students;
- Local governments are responsible for public health services, for managing local hospitals, for investment in local hospitals and for the management and financing of public nursing homes (which are not covered by them statutory insurance scheme).

Self-government (Selbstverwaltung) is an important principle in the German health care system. The government devolves specified powers and duties to certain regulated but self-governing bodies, including sickness funds and physicians' associations, which represent private interest groups, but compulsory membership. Since 1977 an important advisory function regarding rationalisation and efficiency of the health care system has been allocated to the Concerted Action Council in Health Care. This body consists of 64 members from the insurance agencies, the medical professions, employers, labour unions, pharmaceutical industry and politicians. This composition is an indication of the pluralistic character of the German health care system. Private initiative, semi-public organisations and government organisations have divided power in an intricate system of co-operation and negotiations.
The task of transforming the previously state-managed health care system of the former German Democratic Republic into the model of the federal republic requires substantial changes. About 15,000 physicians who settled down as self-employed doctors had to buy new equipment, hire staff and rent offices. The upgrading of hospitals in the "new Länder" will require huge investments in order to meet the standards of those in the western part of the country.

5.3 *Financing of health care*

The following table gives data on the sources of financing of public health in Germany. Data published by the Statistisches Bundesamt reflect all the aspects included in the field of public health. In the data published by BASYS some public health costs have been excluded in order to make their data more suitable for international comparison of health care costs. These excluded costs relate to income compensations in the case of illness and the costs of investments, research and administration. The result is that the role of social security, individual payments and private insurance as sources of health care financing becomes more important.

Table 5.1
Germany: Financial sources, 1990 (percentages of total)

	St. Ba [1]	BASYS
	1990	1990
General taxation	13.3	12.0
Social security	55.6	66.2
Individual payments	7.8	12.9
Private insurance	5.7	7.7
Employers	17.6	1.1
Total	100.0	100.0

1) Statistisches Bundesamt.

5.4 *Insurance structure*

The system of social sickness insurance in Germany is an integrated part of the system of social security and is regulated by law. About 88% of the population is insured in accordance with this system. There is compulsory insurance for employees, the unemployed, pensioners (if sickness fund members in their active life), farmers, handicapped, students and trainees. In principle spouses and children are co-insured.

There is no compulsory insurance for employees who earn more than a fixed amount, and civil servants under special regulations. These two categories can take part voluntarily in the public sickness fund scheme or choose an individual private insurance.

The social sickness insurance is operated by more than 1100 sickness funds, co-ordinated by umbrella organisations at federal level and at state (Land) level:

681 Betriebskrankenkassen (industry and trade)
150 Innungskrankenkassen (skilled labour)

19 Landwirtschaftliche Krankenkassen (agriculture)
Seekrankenkasse (seamen)
Bundesknappschaft (miners)

Moreover there are two kinds of sickness funds, which are not based on professions:
262 Ortskrankenkassen (local sickness funds)
15 Ersatzkassen (voluntarily insured)

The sickness funds are organisations under public law and have regulating power in a structure of self-government (Selbsverwaltung). Autonomous organisations of sickness funds decide on extent and nature of benefits and the height of contributions. Sickness funds are under administrative control of the government. Their bookkeeping is controlled at federal level by the Bundesversicherungsamt and at state level by the Arbeits- und Sozialminister of the Land.

Sickness funds must establish a general assembly, a board and a general secretary. Orts-, Betriebs-, and Innungskrankenkassen have to form a regional organisation in every state, where members are represented. They also form central organisations at federal level (Bundesverbände). Contributions to the sickness funds can vary from 8% in the Betriebskrankenkassen to 16% in the Ortskrankenkassen. This is due to the autonomy of the sickness fund.

Private insurance companies offer complete health care insurance or supplementary insurance for sickness fund members. Almost 10% of the German population is connected with a private insurance company. Premiums are related to the extent of the insurance, age, sex and personal health.

5.4.1 *Sickness funds benefits*

The statutory sickness insurance scheme in Germany covers an extensive package of benefits: ambulatory care by medical doctors and dentists, pharmaceuticals and therapeutic appliances, intramural care, home care and rehabilitation services. Also some preventive treatments and examinations are paid by the sickness funds like dental prevention for youngsters and medical check-ups every two years for persons above the age of 35. Special features of the sickness fund benefits in Germany are payment of the costs of any necessary course of treatment at a health spa (Kurort) and a compensation of 80% of the person's income, if such a benefit is not provided by the employer, for the period of incapacity. Child sickness benefits can be paid to parents in order to compensate income loss while caring for a sick child at home.

After death of the insured person relatives receive a grant (Sterbegeld) as a contribution to the funeral costs. For the compulsory insured services are in kind, but for the voluntary insured costs are reimbursed.

5.4.2 *Cost sharing*

Though the coverage of the sickness funds is said to be generous, Germans also have to pay own contributions for certain health services. If prices of pharmaceuticals are not fixed, everyone older than 19 years must pay 3 DM per prescription. Since 1 January 1992 15 % of the costs of pharmaceuticals with a maximum of 15 DM are borne by the patient. Therapeutic appliances are charged with a co-payment of 10%.

In the case of glasses only a fixed price is paid. Transport of patients requires co-payments of 20 DM. Since 1 January 1991 10 DM per day (for 14 days) must be paid in hospitals (children excluded). In health spas (Kurorten) this amount is 15 DM. In case of orthopaedic jaw operations 20% and for dentures 40% must be contributed.

Insured patients with low incomes are exempted from co-payments and for other categories, too, exceptions have been made, e.g. for therapeutic appliances and pharmaceuticals for children under 18, pregnancy complaints, industrial accidents and impairments due to war, military service and civil protection.

5.5 *Fee and salary structure*

Medical doctors, working in hospitals receive a salary and in the case of private patients a fee-for-service. They are organised in the "Marburger Bund". Their salary is dependent on specialism and seniority.

To be eligible to charge for ambulatory care services doctors must be members of a regional association of physicians. Every year the sickness funds and the regional associations negotiate a global budget, "Gesamtvergütung". The sickness funds transfer the revenues they collect from employers and employees to the regional associations of doctors, which reimburse their members on a fee-for-service basis. For this purpose physicians submit quarterly a list of treatments rendered. The role of the physicians associations as payers is unique for Germany. To stay within budget limits there is a relation between the volume and the amount: the higher the volume, the lower the reimbursement per claim in the next quarter.

This system turned out to be an effective way to control physicians' fees. Doctors whose service patterns differ substantially from the norm are invited to discuss their practices with the regional physicians committee.

Day rates for hospitals are fixed between hospitals and sickness funds on the basis of past cost data. The cost of comparable hospitals and the recommendations of the West German Hospital Association and the Association of Statutory Health Insurance Carriers with regard to efficiency in hospital care must be taken into consideration.

5.6 *Policy developments in health care*

The explosive increase in expenditures on health care caused a strong rise in sickness fund contributions by employers and employees. In connection with the economic problems of the German Unification and the general position of the industry in international competition, drastic reforms became inevitable.

In 1993 the Health Care Structural Reform Act came into force. This act contains measures, directed to immediate cost reduction and measures with structuring effects for health care in the future:

- strict budgeting of sickness fund expenditure for the years 1993–1995 with regard to expenditures incurred by doctors, dentists and hospitals, as well as the administrative costs of the sickness funds. Until 1995 these expenditures may not increase at a greater rate than the salaries of the insured.
- limitation at the level of 1991 of the expenses for pharmaceuticals and physiotherapy.
- limitation of the number of self-employed medical doctors and dentists by means of regional planning.
- reform of the fee structure for self-employed general practitioners and specialists.
- introduction of a positive list of pharmaceuticals, co-payments by the insured and extension of the list of fixed prices.
- lower prices for dentures and a 2-year guarantee for fillings and dentures; improvement of dental prevention.
- introduction of a new day rate system for hospitals, based on
- diagnosis related groups, broken down by wards (standardized treatment on a lump sum basis).
- expansion of day treatment facilities.
- extra financial means for nursing staff.
- reform of the statutory insurance scheme with enlargement of freedom of choice for the insured and standardized payments for sickness funds.
- improvement of the opportunities for mergers of sickness funds.
- equaization of risks among sickness funds due to limit the variance of contribution rates.
- introduction in 1995 of a distinct insurance for nursing care, as well for nursing care at home (1995) as in nursing homes (1996).

The initial effects of the already operational measures of the health Care Structural Reform Act seem to be very positive:

- in 1993 sickness funds expenditure decreased by 1.3% after an increase of 10% in both 1991 and 1992.
- the financing deficit of 9.4 billion DM in 1992 has been replaced by a surplus of 10.4 billion DM in 1993.
- the explosive rise of sickness fund contributions (12.2% in 1992 and 13.4% in 1993) came to an end.

5.7 *Organisation of health care*

5.7.1 *General characteristics*

A conspicuous feature of German health care is the sharp division between ambulatory care and hospital care. In general, hospitals do not offer out patient care. Doctors working in extramural care do not have access to hospital facilities.

Patients are free to choose a general practitioner or visit a self-employed specialist without referral.

About 1400 of the 3500 hospitals are public, owned by federal government, Länder or local authorities. Private hospitals are often owned by religious organisations or by doctors. About half of private hospitals are non-profit based.

Patients are free to choose their doctor. This can be a general practitioner or a specialist in independent practice. For hospital admission the patient needs a referral by an ambulatory care doctor. Sickness fund patients are normally referred to the nearest hospital with suitable facilities. Private patients and selected sickness fund patients can be referred to hospitals outside the area.

5.7.2 *Intramural care*

There are more than 3500 hospitals in Germany, of which about 2200 are defined by law as "Krankenhäuser" and about 1200 as "Vorsorge- und Rehabilitations-einrichtungen". Acute care is mainly provided in general hospitals. Long term care is given in nursing homes and special geriatric department of hospitals.

Acute hospitals, providing standard care, usually have few specialisms: general internal medicine and surgery, supplemented by obstetrics and gynaecology. They provide basic in-patient care. Major hospitals provide care for more than their own region and have more specialist departments.

Central hospitals are frequently university clinics and at the same time teaching hospitals. In general they cover all aspects of medicine and exercise a supra regional and sometimes even a nation-wide care function. Nursing homes and homes for the elderly are provided outside the statutory health insurance system by local authorities and voluntary bodies. They are financed mainly by private expenditure, often supported by social assistance.

Authors like Hurst emphasise the sharp division between hospitals and extramural care and the absence of outpatient facilities in hospitals. German sources indicate ambulatory care provision by hospitals.

5.7.3 *Extramural care in Germany*

5.7.3.1 Medical care

a. *General Remarks*

Extramural medical care in Germany is provided by independent general practitioners and specialists (niedergelassene Ärzte); the vast majority of them (95%) holds a license to treat public sickness fund (PSF-) patients (Vertragsärzte). In Germany, patients are free to choose their doctor. This can be a general practitioner or a specialist. Just recently, a discussion has begun concerning the general practitioner acting as a gatekeeper.

Medical doctors treating PSF-patients are organised in associations, "Kassenärztliche Vereinigungen", which negotiate on remuneration and distribute these among their members, but also exercise responsibilities in the area of quality of praxis. Remuneration is on the basis of quasi-money (points) since the introduction of a budget for ambulatory care. The value of a point can be fixed only at the end of the year, when the total number of points charged by all physicians (and dentists) can be compared to the available budget. The money value of such a point has decreased by up to 25% over the last 2 years due to an increased number of doctors and new regulations. Dramatic financial problems may occur in quite a few practices leading to bankruptcy, especially in new practices with great financing obligations.

b. *Dimensions and types of activity*

In 1994 there were 105,000 Vertragsärzte practising in 75,000 practices. Jointly run practices continuously gain importance; nowadays 1 out of 4 doctors provides his services in such an institution. The average number of employees of a practice varies from 1 to 11, depending mainly on its gross turnover.

Special regulations of minor importance need to be mentioned. In some cases a doctor employed in either a hospital or working in administration may be licensed to treat PSF-patients, if there is a substantial shortage in his region and speciality. Such "ermächtigte Ärzte" made up 11,000 in 1993; the total of all physicians practising in ambulatory care being 126,000, therefore.

c. *Regulations*

An increasing oversupply of physicians in ambulatory care has been found using standard quotas of physician density. Out of 544 planning regions 43 to 70% are judged as oversupplied, depending on the specific medical speciality. In such oversupplied regions no additional licenses to treat sickness fund patients are issued. The total number of available licenses in the non-restricted regions is about 8.000.

d. *Structure of providers*

The physician density varies per regions – in general, it is lower in the new Länder – with the values ranging from 106.4 per 100,000 inhabitants (Sachsen-Anhalt) to 164.0 (Berlin) with an overall average of 131.0. (all values 1993). The average net increase of the number of physicians in ambulatory practice was 2.4% (1,200 doctors) in 1993 after a temporary up in 1992 due to organisational changes.

The average age of physicians in ambulatory care has decreased dramatically over the last 20 years. Median age is now 44 years. Hospital doctors are in general younger, however. The overall percentage of female doctors is 31% (1994), with great regional variations in the old Länder (21–37%); in the New Länder it is substantially higher (57%).

41.7% of all Vertragsärzte provide general practitioner's services, although it has to be mentioned that a clear cut medical education for becoming a general practitioner does not exist in Germany. Quite a few medical specialities enable to settle as a general practitioner – e.g. internal medicine, paediatrics – in addition to those directly qualifying like "Allgemeinmedizin" or "praktischer Arzt".

58.3% of all physicians in ambulatory care provide specialists' services: the main fields of service are internal medicine (14.1% of all physicians), gynaecologists (8.6%), paediatrics (5.3%). In 1993, ambulatory services have increased specifically in the fields of psychiatric care and surgery.

e. *Turnover, Income, Equipment*

The average turnover of all practices with PSF-patients was 365,000 DM in 1993, the median value being 280,000 DM. The turnover with non-PSF-patients (private health insurance) is estimated at 44,000 DM in 1993, the total turnover being close to 400,000 DM.

Turnover varies greatly with medical speciality. Average values for PSF-patients alone range from 280,000 DM (g.p's) to 860,000 DM (radiologists); the high values concentrate on specialities using technical equipment. Ambulatory practices in general are well equipped and have ample access to most diagnostic services. Even scanners and magneto-resonance devices are included. In the last couple of years, the annual increase of the number of new devices has been substantially higher in ambulatory care than in stationary care.

5.7.3.2 Dental care

a. *General Remarks*

Dental care in Germany is provided by independent dentists, the vast majority of whom holds a license to treat public sickness fund (PSF-) patients (Vertragszahnärzte). Values for the percentage of Vertragszahnärzte in all practising dentists vary with regions; in the New Länder it is generally higher (88%) than in the Old ones (81%). In Germany, patients are free to choose their dentist. This holds true also for dental surgeons.

Dentists treating PSF-patients are organised in associations, "Kassenzahn-ärzt-liche Vereinigungen", which negotiate on remuneration and distribute these among their members, but also exercise responsibilities in the area of quality of praxis. Remuneration is on the basis of quasi-money (points) since the introduction of a budget for ambulatory care. The value of a point can be fixed only at the end of the year, when the total number of points charged by all physicians (and dentists) can be compared to the available budget. The money value of such a point is generally higher than with physicians, due to a different remuneration scheme.

b. *Dimensions and types of activity*

In 1994 there were 49,050 Vertragszahnärzte in 46,100 practices, i.e. 12% of all dentists provided their services in a jointly run practice. 2,320 of all Vertrags-zahnärzte provide only jaw surgery services. 83% of all practising dentists treat PSF-patients in own practices.

c. *Regulations*

An increasing oversupply of dentists was found using standard quotas of dentist density. In 1994 out of 1,966 planning regions an average of 15% were judged as oversupplied, with regional values ranging up to 64% in Berlin. With respect to jaw surgery 3% of 617 planning regions are judged as over-supplied.

d. *Structure of providers*

The dentist density varies by regions – in general, it is higher in the new Länder – with the values ranging from 47 per 100,000 inhabitants (Saarland) to 79 (Berlin) with an overall average of 60. (all values 1993). The average net increase of the number of physicians in ambulatory practice is 2.4% (1,200 doctors).

The average age of dentist in ambulatory care has decreased. Median age is now 40 years. The overall percentage of female dentists is 33% (1994), with a great difference between the Old Länder (25%) and the New Länder (58%).

4.7% of all Vertragszahnärzte provide only jaw surgery services, the number of jaw surgeons increased more rapidly than the one of other dentists in the past 3 years.

The average number of employees of a dentist's practice is 5 in the old Länder and 4 in the new Länder. In 1 out of 6 practices the owner employs an additional dentist (not to be mixed up with jointly run practices).

e. *Turnover, Income, Equipment*

The average gross turnover of the practice with PSF-patients is 678,000 DM in the old Länder, 506,000 DM in the New Länder and 635,000 DM altogether. The turnover with non-PSF-patients (private health insurance and private co-payments) is estimated at more than 60,000 DM in 1993, the total turnover being close to 700,000 DM.

5.7.3.3 *Pharmacists*

a. *General Remarks*

Pharmacists provide their services either in public pharmacies or in hospital pharmacies. The latter take care of pharmaceutical supply of one or more hospitals (joint hospital pharmacy) and don't serve individual customers.

Public pharmacies supply:

- pharmaceuticals, which require the prescription of a doctor (verschreibungspflichtige Arzneimittel);
- pharmaceuticals, which don't require such a prescription but are only allowed to be sold by pharmacies (apothekenpflichtige Arzneimittel – OTC);
- other pharmaceuticals (freiverkäufliche Arzneimittel – OTC);
- other products like body care and cosmetics (sonstiges Sortiment).

Pharmacists are also organised in associations with a mandatory membership (Apothekenkammer). These organisations take care of education, association politics, they do, however, not negotiate with health insurance funds in a comparable legal context as the physicians' or dentists' associations do.

b. *Dimensions and types of activity*

In Germany there were 20,903 pharmacies in 1994, 18,197 in the Old Länder and 2,706 in the New. In the New Länder this number has increased since reunification by 45.5% with the pharmacy density still being substantially lower there. Values for this density range from 16.5 to 18.6 per 100,000 in the New Länder and from 26.8 to 34.1 in the Old Länder. It must be expected that density values in the New Länder will approach those in the Old in the very near future. Furthermore, the density in the Old Länder did not change noticeably since 1990, leading to the assumption that the actual value is economically balanced.

c. *Regulations*

The retail prices for pharmaceuticals are legally fixed (Festpreise) and calculated by adding a constant wholesale and retails sales surcharge (percentage) on the producer's sales price. Discounts given to pharmacies by gross sellers are not allowed to be given to the customer. Pharmaceuticals to be remunerated by the health insurance funds are given a 5% discount. The retail seller's share of the retail price varies between 33.5% and 17%, mainly by the amount ordered.

Remuneration for pharmaceuticals is strictly regulated. In 1989 a fixed prices for the group of "comparable pharmaceuticals" was introduced. This lead to a considerable price decrease of original products and to an increase of market share of generic pharmaceuticals. In 1996 those comparable pharmaceuticals made up 75% of the total turnover with pharmaceuticals. For the non-regulated pharmaceuticals a co-payment was introduced in 1992 (GSG). This co-payment made up 3 DM, 5 DM or 7 DM, depending on the package size.

In 1993 the responsibility for cost containment was shifted to the physicians in ambulatory care. With a fixed budget for all prescribed pharmaceuticals any excess of the budget is compensated for by an equally high cut of the budget for ambulatory care, i.e. the money value of the „point" (see above) decreases. This lead to a 10.5% decrease in prescriptions in 1993 and a 15.3% decrease in the respective pharmaceutical expenditures. Only 91% and 95% of the budget were used in1993 and 1994 respectively.

d. *Structure of providers*

The number of employees in all pharmacies (owners excluded) totalled 124,230 in 1994 with 105,856 in the Old Länder. The average number of employees in the Old Länder raised slightly from 5.4 to 5.8 with the last 10 years, in the New Länder it has decreased from 10 to 6.8 since 1989.

In the Old Länder about 33% of the pharmacy personnel (owners included) are pharmacists, 33% are pharmaceutical helpers (3 years of vocational training) and 33% are other personnel often in administration.

86% of all licensed pharmacists work in public pharmacies, 4% in hospital pharmacies and 10% in other professions.

e. *Turnover, Income, Equipment*

The average turnover of a pharmacy was 2.1 Mill. DM or 540 DM per inhabitant. The percentage share of turnover broken down by types of pharmaceuticals (see above) is:

- verschreibungspflichtige Arzneimittel: 61.0%,
- apothekenpflichtige Arzneimittel: 30.5%,
- freiverkäufliche Arzneimittel: 2.0%,
- sonstiges Sortiment: 6.5%.

66% of the pharmacy's turnover is remunerated by public sickness funds, 33% is paid for by private households, either as the legally required co-payment or as OTC purchases.

5.7.3.4 *Paramedical care*

a. *General Remarks*

In Germany, various forms of ambulatory paramedical care exist. Substantial information is available only for those negotiating with PSF and being licensed by them.

As a general rule it may be stated, that paramedical services for PSF-patients are remunerated, if prescribed by a licensed physician (Vertragsarzt) or following a hospital stay. For clarification it is stated, that under the label of paramedical care the following services are subcategorised in Germany:

- midwives,
- non-medical practitioners (Heilpraktiker) – 3 years of training
- physiotherapists
- speech therapists
- ergo therapists
- psychotherapists,
- others (dieticians, health advisors, chiropodists [medizinische Fußpfleger], music therapists)

b. *Dimensions and types of activity*

Paramedical care is a sector of growing importance within ambulatory health care in Germany. Expenditures for such services have grown since 1970 with a rate twice as high as the one of total health expenditures. The number of practices raised by 161% since 1970, the number of employees by 290% (for comparison: the respective numbers for the overall health sector are 43% and 120%)

Density is 5.2 per 100,000 for midwives (range from 3.6 in Northrhine-Westfalia to 8.2 in Schleswig-Holstein), 11.9 for non-medical practitioners (range from 10.1 in Rhineland-Palatinate to 20.5 in Berlin), 39.5 for physiotherapists (range from 25.7 in Berlin to 27.8 in Northrhine-Westfalia), 3.4 for speech therapists, 0.5 for ergotherapists, and 8.8 for psychotherapists.

All above numbers are from 1990 and cover only the Old Länder. In the New Länder paramedical care is growing, density values are judged to be considerable lower. The numbers are restricted to provided ambulatory paramedical care.

c. *Regulations*

In general all such services are directly remunerated by PSF, if prescribed by a Vertragsarzt with the exemption of non-medical practitioners, whose services are non-remunerable with PSF and have to be paid by the patients themselves.

d. *Structure of providers*

Very little is known about the size and number of employees of such paramedical practices. By the type of service one has to assume that in general these practices are small, often a 1-person institution.

e. *Turnover, Income, Equipment*

The total expenditure on paramedical services was 8 Bill DM in 1992. A further breakdown by type of care is not feasible, as the average turnover is expected to vary between categories, and as expenditures cannot be broken down any further.

5.7.3.5 Home nursing and home care [1)]

a. *General Remarks*

In Germany, several types of organisation are involved in providing ambulatory nursing care and household help. They are referred to in general as "ambulante sozialpflegerische Dienste" (organisations for ambulatory social and nursing care):

- Gemeindekrankenstationen;
- Haus- und Familienpflegestationen;
- Sozialstationen;
- Mobile Soziale Hilfsdienste.

Social care and welfare services are provided mainly by independent charity associations, but also by self-organised groups and – gaining continuously importance since the introduction of the Public Nursing Care Insurance (PNI) – by private business. Home nursing is provided by so-called "Gemeindekranken-pflege-stationen" (organisations for home nursing only) and increasingly by "Sozialstationen" (providing a broad range of ambulatory services, including home nursing and home help services.

In the provision of services, a quite important legal distinction is made between "Grundpflege" (helping the patient with basic needs including ADL-activities) and "Behandlungspflege" (specialised, technical nursing procedures). The two types of care are generally carried out by "Krankenschwestern" (nurses with 3 years of training), and with the exception of technical nursing by "Krankenschwester-helferinnen" (2 years of training) and "Altenpflegerinnen".

First contacts between patient and home nurse are often initiated by the family or neighbours, but also by general practitioners or by hospitals, which contact the "Sozialstation" a few days before discharging a patient. Officially, the assessment is done by either a physician, whose orders are needed for reimbursement of home nursing by the health insurance funds. Physicians however, closely co-operate with head nurses of Social Stations in assessing patients. Usually, the head nurse of the "Sozialstation" also decides which level of expertise is needed and who is going to deliver the care. Normally, care is given by the nurse serving the specific area in which the patient lives. Since doctor's orders are needed for reimbursement, the assessment forms (which are used in "Sozialstationen") are adapted to this.

Since the introduction of PNI the process of defining a person as "needing nursing care" has changed. For obtaining funds from the PNI it is necessary to be declared eligible by a doctor of the "Sozialmedizinischer Dienst der Krankenkas-sen (SDK)", the physicians board of PNI.

Home help services are provided by three types of organisations. "Traditional" home help services are provided by „Haus- und Familiepflegestationen" and by "Sozialstationen".

Additional home help services mainly for elderly people are provided also by „Mobilen sozialen Hilfsdienste". They provide services such as meals-on-wheels and cleaning services, which enable the elderly (and chronically ill) to stay in their own homes, instead of being admitted to nursing homes or old people's homes. The traditional "Haus- und Familienpflege" provides temporary care for families or individuals at home. This care includes basic nursing care, pedagogical and psychological care, and homemaking services. Typical of traditional home help services is its diversity as far as the provision of services is concerned. Clients are families with children as well as elderly people. "Mobile soziale Hilfsdienste" provide:

- information and advice on social and other ambulatory services;
- homemaking services (help with cooking meals, doing the dishes, tidying up and so on);
- so-called „Betreuungsdienste" (keep the elderly company, help with correspondence, accompany clients to their doctor and so on);
- some basic nursing, such as helping clients getting dressed;
- shopping and cleaning services.

Clients are predominantly people over 65 years of age, women, widow(er)s, living on their own. Almost half of the clients have a "Schwerbehinderten-ausweis", a document indicating disability.

PNI started payments for ambulatory nursing in 1995. 1,1 million people are estimated to need one of the 3 levels of care:

category 1: "erheblich Pflegebedürftige", people who need help with at least two activities of daily living once a day and who need home help services several times a week.

category 2: "Schwerpflegebedürftige", people who need help with activities of daily living at least three times a day and who need home help services several times a week.

category 3: "Schwerstpflegebedürftige", people who need help with activities of daily living 24 hours a day and who need home help services several times a week.

b. *Dimensions and types of activity*

In 1993, in West-Germany there were 2,061 organisations for the separate provision of either home nursing (Gemeindekrankenpflegestationen) or of „traditional" home help services (Haus- und Familienpflegestationen), providing home help mainly in families with children under 12, where the mother is hospitalised, has been discharged from hospital or is temporarily incapable of attending to the home and the family for other reasons. The number of these separate organisations had decreased with about 30% (there used to be 2,919 in 1990). At the same time, the number of organisations for home nursing and home help (Sozialstationen) and of mobile soziale Hilfsdienste (providing help at home mainly for the elderly in contrast to the „traditional" home help services) had grown, from 2,869 in 1990 to 3,295 in 1993. In the former GDR, the total number of 894 organisations for home help and nursing care consisted predominantly of Sozialstationen, of which there were 666 in 1993.

Though it is possible to give a general outline of home nursing and home help services in Germany, it should be noted that the details of the organisation of home care vary greatly throughout the country. The regulations determined in federal law are, of course, the same throughout the republic, but since the implementation of legal guidelines is left to the Länder, the actual care provision differs regionally.

c. *Structure of providers*

In 1996 the number for licensed ambulatory care units in Germany was 9,914 (estimate), meaning 12.4 per 100,000 inhabitants. It should be mentioned, that additional 1,350 units provide day care, 325 night care and 3,220 short term care, which will most likely be treated as semistationary care in legal terms.

The size of the population that is served by a „Sozialstation" varies between 12,000 and 50,000 depending on its size and the degree of urbanisation. Usually, „Sozialstationen" in urban areas serve a larger number of inhabitants.

Though the market for home nursing is dominated by non-profit organisations, in recent years a growing number of nurses have decided to work freelance or have developed for-profit nursing organisations. For-profit organisations have developed mainly in urban areas. E.G. in Hamburg 60% of home nursing are delivered by for-profit providers."

5.7.3.6 *Extramural mental health care services*

a. *General Remarks*

Extramural mental health care facilities were introduced to the traditional intramural services in the 60es and 70es. In general it holds true that the quantitative importance of these services is lower than in other countries (e.g. Great Britain). Furthermore, after quite a number of feasibility studies, a variety of services and organisational forms have been developed in the different Länder, due to different legislative initiatives.

Extramural mental health services are provided by mental specialists (medical specialists), hospital ambulances of psychiatric hospitals, sociopsychiatric services (see PHO) and providers of parademical care (psychotherapists – see above). Ambulatory medical health treatment is often supported by activities enabling patients to live on their own such as guided housing, therapeutically guided living groups etc.

b. *Dimensions and types of activity*

The density of mental specialist per 100,000 varies between 2.5 (Saxonia) and 21.2 (Baden-Württemberg) with an overall total of 5.2 – using the definition of density provided be the KBV (doctors medical association). In some areas an oversupply is stated already as a target value of 1 specialist to 17,348 inhabitants has been introduced in 1993 (target density: 5.8 per 100,000).

The density of qualified personnel in psychiatric hospital ambulances per 100,000 cannot be provided. It is known, however, that such ambulances on average have 4.12 employees, among them 1.09 physicians.

Sociopsychiatric services have an average density of 1.9 per 100,000 (data for Baden-Württemberg 1992 only).

The density numbers for paramedical services are 10.0 (psychotherapists) and .88 (ergotherapists) in 1994.

5.7.3.7 Extramural centres for alcohol and drugs addicts

There are no specific services for alcohol or drug addicts. People needing such services (alcoholism) have to address a physician or may be granted a withdrawal cure. Alcohol addicts are often members in self-organised associations with a non-profit character (like Anonymous Alcoholics, Blue Cross etc.).

For drug addicts special programs exist in metropolitan services (like methadone substitution or the „clean needle program"); these programs run under the auspices of the municipal or county social office rather than the health office, however.

5.7.3.8 Ambulance services and patient transport

a. *General Remarks*

In Germany, the "Länder" or subregional bodies are responsible for the legally required "sufficient degree of infrastructure" for the transport of patients. These bodies pay for investment and training of personnel – like in the hospital sector – whereas running cost have to be born by the users via health insurance funds or private health insurance.

Emergency centres are set up regionally. For the most part, the actual provision of services is performed by private (non-profit) organisations such as the Red

Cross, the "Malteser Hilfdienst", the "Arbeiter-Samariterbund" and the "Johanniter-Unfallhilfe". In addition, the fire brigade plays an important role, especially in the event of an emergency.

There is a strict division between ambulance service (both emergencies and regular transport) and other forms of patient transport.

Ambulance service is carried out by specially trained personnel using special means of transport. They have at their disposal the use of helicopters, aeroplanes ("Flugrettung"), ambulances ("Krankentransportwagen" or KTW), emergency ambulances ("Rettungswagen" or RTW) and medically equipped emergency ambulances ("Notarztwagen" or NAW). RTW's and NAW's are used in the case of accidents. KTW's are for the purpose of transport on request.

Emergency transport is initiated and the suitable means of transport chosen by the emergency control office (Rettungsleitstelle), the nearest of which can be reached from everywhere dialling 110. There is always one single emergency control office in charge for a defined region. It can be at a fire or a county office or an emergency health station providing 24 hour service.

Furthermore, there is yet another, "non-public", form of ambulance service, used by hospitals for the transport between intramural institutes. Hospitals may use their own ambulances for this purpose, or call in the services of ambulances from other organisations. The costs of this type of transport is allowed for in the hospital fees.

Patient transport, defined as such, relates to the general means of transport without specially trained personnel, such as taxis. A doctor's certificate is required in order to be considered for compensation. In some cases compensation is paid to people with insufficient financial means of their own.

b. *Dimensions and types of activity*

The number of emergency transports per 100,000 (RTW) varies regionally from 1,584 in Baden-Württemberg to 8,444 in Hamburg with an average of 2,786. The number of emergency transports with an emergency doctor (NAW) varies from 938 in Schleswig-Holstein to 3,155 in Thuringia with an average of 1,576. The number of non-emergency ambulance services per 100,000 (KTW) varies between 3,220 (Schleswig-Holstein) and 8,912 (Berlin) with an average of 5,938.

The number of patient transports is unknown. Using expenditure data of PSF and assuming an average charge of 20 DM per transport one would end up with more than 30,000 such transports per 100,000 population.

c. *Regulations*

Any form of ambulance service or patient transport requires a physician's „necessity certificate", comparable to a prescription. The type of transport judged necessary by the physician is remunerated. In cases of emergency where such certificates are not at hand, it is in the value judgement of the sickness fund on whether or not a remuneration will be granted. If an emergency number is called (110) and the person in charge send an emergency ambulance car after interviewing the caller, costs will be remunerated.

These regulations are also valid with respect to patient transport. Taking a cab to see a doctor in his practice is running a risk in case this physician will not certify the necessity. In this case the patient should have used public transport or his own car. Remuneration can be granted still, however, in case of personal need (insufficient financial means) on a voluntary basis.

d. *Structure of providers*

Ambulance services are provided by Feuerwehr (fire department), the only fiscal organisation on municipal or county level and by 4 non-profit organisations. The percentage shares for emergency and non-emergency transports are 38% and 59% (Red Cross), 5% and 6.6% (Malteser Hilfsdienst), 7.3% and 12% (Arbeiter-Samariterbund), 8.6% and 6.4% (Johanniter-Unfallhilfe), and 41.1% and 15.8% (Feuerwehr).

In Germany there are altogether 442 Rettungsleitstellen (emergency control offices) and 2,123 Rettungswachen (emergency units with 24 hour service). The number of emergency ambulance cars is 3,451, the number of ambulance cars is 4,782 with a total density of 10.3 transport units per 100,000.

e. *Turnover, Income, Equipment*

Running emergency transport and patients transport is expensive due to the high fixed costs emerging from 24 hour availability. Public sickness funds spend 76 Million DM on airbound ambulance services, 520 Mill DM on transports with emergency cars and 470 Mill DM on transports with emergency doctor cars. Patient transport (taxis) costs 483 Mill. DM. All data are 1992 and cover around 88% of the population – PSF-members.

Total expenditures for all forms of emergency and non-emergency ambulances as well as for patient transports are estimated at 3.4 Bill DM in 1992.

5.7.3.9 *Medical laboratories*

a. *General Remarks*

Describing the situation with ambulatory medical and dental laboratories is quite crucial. Lab services initiated by g.p's and medical specialists may either be provided within the practice of the initiating physician or it may be purchased on the market – with some strict regulations holding true.

With respect to dentists lab services have to be kept separate from any activities concerning full or partial tooth replacement. The first is, in general, of minor importance and is treated exactly the way as with physicians.

The latter is provided not by dentists, but by people with a specific vocational training „Zahntechniker" (dental technician). Those services are purchased from „dental labs" owned and run by such a „Zahntechniker", if the dentist doesn't employ one or more of such „Zahntechniker" in his/her practice.

b. *Dimensions and types of activity*

The number of lab communities is not exactly known, nor is its regional distributions. The number used to be around 1,000 in the Old Länder in the seventies and is estimated to have decreased to no more than 200-250 in 1995 (Germany) due to economic pressures (economies of scale). We do not know of any significant amount of lab services either exported or imported in the area of medical laboratories.

The number of institutions providing very specific, seldom or expensive lab tests like chromosome or hormone testing is by far smaller (less than 40).

Artificial teeth and other dental prostheses, however, are produced by a great number of small enterprises (Gesundheitshandwerk) with 1 through 10 employees. The total number of such dental prostheses providers was7,017 in 1995 (official statistics). Rumours go, that a growing number of dental prostheses are purchased in the far east (Hongkong), with no details known, however.

c. *Regulations*

In order to have a lab service remunerated by PSF this service has to be personally provided by physician holding a license for treating PSF-patients. His/her speciality need not be laboratory medicine, however.

This prerequisite led to the system of „Laborgemeinschaften" (lab communities), jointly owned by a number of physicians in ambulatory care. The business-law construction used is the one of BGB-Gemeinschaft (Civilian Law Community) in which all members jointly own and bear the business risk of the enterprise. Those labs work in their own rooms with their own personnel.

Theoretically, lab services could also be purchased at a hospital; this would, however, require the physician in charge of the hospital lab to hold the status of „ermächtigter Arzt" (see above). It is virtually non-existent.

d. *Structure of providers*

Lab services are either provided with means of the physician's or dentist's own practice. These services are estimated to be between 10 and 20% of all medical lab services (physicians) and between 10 and 15% of all dental lab services. The rest is purchased from other providers.

e. *Turnover, Income, Equipment*

The average turnover of a lab community can be estimated at less than 18.9 Mill DM in 1994 using the respective expenditure data and the number of providers. As it is common knowledge that the prices the lab charges the physician with, are lower than the remuneration he receives for it (it pays to have the lab services outsourced.), the real turnover values cannot be provided, only the value of the remunerated equivalent.

With respect to labs providing dental prostheses the average turnover was close to 850,000 DM in 1994, due to the smaller size of those enterprises.

The total expenditures for ambulatory lab services are 4.683 Bill. DM for medical labs, 3 Mill. DM for dentists' medical labs and 10.967 Bill. DM for dental labs (prostheses). Out of the latter, 50% are purchased from the market and 50% are produced by dental technicians in a dentist's practice. The average turnover of a dentist's practice with their own production of prostheses is 780,000 DM in 1994.

5.7.3.10 Municipal or county public health offices

a. *General Remarks*

Municipal or county public health offices (PHO) is the German equivalent of the Public Health Service in the Anglo-Saxon countries. Its quantitative importance is by far smaller, however. This has not always been the case; the decrease of the PHO's importance is strongly related with the role of PHO in the Third Reich's genocide – enabled by the concentration of both health-police and health-prevention elements in the Stratification Bill 0f 1936.

After the Second World War PHO in East and West Germany developed in quite different ways. The GDR there was a strong publicly organised health care systems, whereas in the FRG the importance of PHO continually decreased, mostly due to decreasing funds.

Since the 70s and – in the New Länder since 1989 – a down-sized PHO has been developed. Environmental surveillance has been moved to the new environment offices, health prevention to the physicians in ambulatory care. Traditionally, in Germany existed the 3 column paradigm: ambulatory care, stationary care and public health services. This is no longer valid because of the respective financial shares.

b. *Dimensions and types of activity*

In 4 out of 16 Länder PHO is organised at county level, in 7 it is solely the responsibility of the local (municipal) bodies, in 3 both forms exist parallel, and in Hamburg and Berlin PHO is organised at the level of town districts. Special tasks like virological, microbiological and chemical examinations are often performed by specific offices (outsourcing).

Supervision of PHO is either with the Land Health Ministry (14) or a Land Public Health Office (2). At the federal level supervision is performed by the Robert-Koch-Institute, the former Federal Public Health Office.

Activities of PHO in the broadest sense include „Gesundheitsvorsorge" (health prevention with education, information and counselling), "Gesundheits-förderung" (health fostering), „Gesundheitsschutz" (prevention of epidemics, supervision of especially endangered groups, vaccination and food control) and „Gesundheitshilfe und -fürsorge" (health aid and welfare with school and youth health, support for the handicapped, socio-psychiatric services).

c. *Structure of providers*

Nowadays PHO is a mixtum compositum of surveillance of notifiable diseases, school health, school dental health, social work, psychological counselling and offers for drug addicts (e.g. methadone substitution). PHO is legally regulated by Länder legislation and varies considerably among them. Since 1980 4 Länder have detailed the PHO's responsibilities in new Laws.

The personnel of PHO is structured following this variety of tasks. Physicians and dentists make up 22% and 5%, assistants of the various forms 22%, social workers of various categories 18% and administrators and other personnel 28%. In some PHO there are present up to 37 different qualifications. The office head has still to be a physician, however. Training for being a PHO doctor (Amtsarzt) takes 6 months and follows the regular specialists education (Weiterbildung). In the past the difference between the income of PHO doctors and physicians providing ambulatory care was so great, that only a specific group of physicians applied for PHO jobs. Often not all vacancies could be filled. With the continuing oversupply of physicians (see above) situation has improved, however.

d. *Turnover, Income, Equipment*

The total share of expenditures for PHO in all health expenditures declined continuously from 1.2% in 1970 to 0.8% in 1994. The often heard critique of underfunding is obviously substantiated. It is expected, however, that necessary changes and adaptations will result in a reduction of responsibilities rather than in an increased funding.

5.8 *Preventive health care in Germany*

All patients above the age of 35 have a check-up every two years for early detection, primarily of coronary and circulatory diseases. Screening programmes for cancer and child welfare are available for every insured person. Public health services are provided mainly by local government. Such services include control of infectious diseases, health education, mother and baby care, school health services and environmental protection. At regional level there are offices for occupational safety and health protection, food control offices and environmental protection offices.

5.9 *Medical goods in Germany*

Medical goods include two categories: the category of pharmaceuticals and the category of therapeutic appliances.

5.9.1 *Pharmaceuticals*

Pharmaceuticals are divided in categories of therapeutic effectiveness, for which different co-payments are fixed. A negative list has been introduced, consisting of pharmaceuticals like cough medicines and painkillers, for which no compensation is given from the age of eighteen. If prices of pharmaceuticals are not fixed, everyone older than 19 years must pay 3 DM per prescription.

Since 1 January 1992 15 % of the costs of pharmaceuticals with a maximum of 15 DM are borne by the patient.

Insured patients with low incomes are exempted from co-payments and for other categories, too, exceptions have been made, e.g. for therapeutical appliances and pharmaceuticals for children under 18, pregnancy complaints, industrial accidents and impairments due to war, military service and civil protection.

5.9.2 *Therapeutic appliances*

In Germany a very large package of therapeutic appliances is included in the health accounts, ranging from glasses to medico-technological devices.

5.10 *Other services in Germany*

Other services consist of activities that in general are not being defined as health care in a strict sense, but of activities of which the costs are adopted in the national health accounts of many countries.

The category other services in Germany consists a/o. of occupational & social rehabilitation and income compensation and specific financial support (in case of illness or disability). The education of health care professionals is only partially included (non-university education), as is health research. All expenditures in the field of health administration are also included in the health accounts with the exception of the central government expenditures.

Note

[1] This paragraph is derived from literature no. 13.

6. Country profile: France

6.1 Introduction

The exchange of information in the network of experts facilitated the production of the "country profiles", which are meant to provide:

- a quick introduction to the organisation and administration of the health care systems of the participating countries;
- an exploration of the boundaries of the health care systems;
- a preliminary determination of place and functions of health care;
- an overview of the main policy developments;
- a contribution to transparency, a necessary condition for international comparison.

The country profiles contain information on health care administration, financing, policy developments and the organisation of health care. This information was brought together in the two phases of the project "international comparison of health care data".

In the first phase (1994–1995) the boundaries of the national health care systems were explored. Also general characteristics of health care administration, financing, policy developments and health care organisation were described.

Detailed quantitative data became available on intramural health care. The expression "intramural health care" proved to be a typically Dutch one. Intramural health care is by and large equal to in-patient health care or stationary care. The description used (see Annex 2.4) is health care for patients formally admitted for a period of more than 24 hours and/or institutionalised treatment for a substantial part of the day (or night).

In the second phase of the project (1996–1997) more detailed data were collected on extramural care, preventive health care, medical goods and other services. Also attention was paid to an update of the determination of the boundaries of national health care systems.

Also the expression "extramural health care" proved to be a typically Dutch one. Extramural health care is described as health care provided on a non-residential basis by medical and paramedical professionals or by specialised organisations in home care or home nursing (for a complete description see Annex 2.4).

At the start of the project the intention was to provide country profiles for all the sectors of care described in this report. This goal was not reached. Especially

information on the topic of "other services" is lacking. To a lesser extent the same holds true for the topic of "medical goods".

6.2 Aspects of general administration of health care

In France the right to health care is laid down in the Constitution. Within the centralised governmental system, health care belongs to the responsibilities of the Ministry of Social Affairs, Health and Cities. This Ministry executes control of the health insurance schemes, provides grants and approves the level of doctors' fees and the prices of pharmaceuticals. The 22 regions and 100 departments are all involved to a certain extent in financing and delivering health care. In the regions and departments a director of health and a medical inspector are responsible for the public health care system and the public hospitals.

The main responsibility at regional level is to plan health care and social amenities through the imposition of annual budget controls or a revision of the "health care map", which establishes the number of hospital beds and sets standards for the distribution of expensive high-tech equipment. Departments are responsible for controlling public hospital facilities operating within the public sector. Municipalities play a role in the field of health care in the context of social services.

Despite the great influence of public authorities part of the health care is delivered by non-public hospitals (1/3 of hospital beds), self-employed general practitioners, specialists, home nurses and other professionals. Also in the field of sickness insurance private organisations (non-profit and for-profit) play a role in financing health care.

6.3 Financing of health care

Table 6.1
France: Financial sources, 1980, 1993 (percentages of total) [1]

	France	
	1980	1993
General taxation	2.9	0.8
Social security	76.5	73.9
Individual payments [2]	15.6	19.0
Mutuelles [3]	5.0	6.3
Total	100.0	100.0

Source: SESI.
1) Curative serices and medical goods.
2) Including private insurance.
3) Complementary insurance.

The Service des Statistiques, des Etudes et des Systèmes d'Information (SESI) in Paris observes a decreasing significance of government financing from 2.9% in 1980 to 0.9% in 1993. Also the percentual share of social security has diminished from 76.5% in 1980 to 73.9% in 1993. On the other hand individual payments and expenditures by the Mutuelles have risen substantially in the course of time.

6.4 *Insurance structure*

Social security is built on four pillars in France:

"Régime général":
- Assurance Maladie (sickness insurance)
- Branche Famille (supplementary family benefits)
- Assurance Vieillesse (old age benefits)

and out of the "régime général:
- Assurance Chômage (benefits for the unemployed)

The sickness insurance fulfils two objectives:
- to meet the medical and ancillary health care expenses incurred by the patient.
- to provide the contributor with a replacement income in case of absence of work or sick-leave.

The social security system is funded by compulsory contributions related to income and shared between employers (70%) and employees (30%). A national central agency (Caisse Nationale d'Assurance Maladie, CNAM) gathers all the contributions collected at local level. Funds are then dispersed to local agencies according to risk. Sickness insurance, covering 99% of the population, is divided into a number of "regimes". The "régime général" is the scheme for salaried people. About 80% of the French population is covered by this scheme. Other schemes include a regime for the self-employed and salaried farmers (9%) and one for the self-employed (6%). Benefits of these schemes are less comprehensive and there are higher rates of co-payment.

The rest of the population is covered by one of about 15 special schemes, with minor advantages for specific sections of the labour force (civil servants etc.). Premiums vary according to the sector in which people are employed and also relate to income. Government pays the insurance for the handicapped and special groups of unemployed.

The national agency (CNAM) is responsible for the co-ordination between 16 regional and 123 local sickness funds and negotiates with professional syndicates in health care. Regional funds negotiate on hospital fees and tariffs. Local sickness funds take care of the administration of the insured and benefits.

In addition to compulsory insurance 87% of the population take out optional supplementary insurance. Private insurance can be divided into profit and non-profit organisations. The latter, "mutuelles" play an important role in French health care. They cover compulsory co-payments and risks not included in the sickness funds.

6.4.1 *Sickness funds benefits*

In order to exercise his rights the insured person must have worked for a certain period and he must have paid sufficient contributions. Also he must be registered with the administrative organ concerned. In the case of loss of his position as insured a person is entitled to sickness fund benefits for a period of twelve months.

In first instance cost of health care services are paid by the patient. These costs are reimbursed afterwards. Reimbursements will always be lower than the costs paid. In the case of industrial accidents or professional diseases the insurance will pay the providers of care directly. Reimbursements are paid for the services of the general practitioner, surgeon, dentist, pharmacist, hospital and nursing home. Costs for rehabilitation, transport and housing for the disabled are also reimbursed.

6.4.2 *Cost sharing*

Co-payments are very common in France. The government has fixed contributions for every kind of service (ticket modérateur). For the service by medical doctors patients pay a legally fixed 30%. The same applies to specialist outpatient treatment, laboratory tests (40%) and X-rays. For the first 30 days of stay in a hospital a forfeit of 55 FF per day has to be paid.

With regard to pharmaceuticals there are differences as to the urgency. Essential drugs are reimbursed completely. Others require co-payments of 35 or 65% or even 100 %. Dental and ophthalmologic care are reimbursed as other medical treatments. Transport costs also are only partially (65%) reimbursed. For dental prostheses, glasses, contact lenses, optical and acoustical aids partial reimbursement is possible after previous agreement with the sickness fund. Other therapeutic appliances are exempted from co-payments.

6.5 *Fee and salary structure*

General practitioners in independent practice and self-employed specialists receive fees for their service. In the sickness fund scheme there is a general regulation on fees, the so-called "nomenclature'. This "nomenclature" consists of three parts:

1. a list of over 4000 procedures grouped under about 50 alpha-numeric codes (or "key letters");
2. a relative value scale for each procedure;
3. a set of monetary multipliers for the alpha-numeric codes.

The doctor charges for the number of points under each alphanumeric code, which contributes to medical secrecy. The list and the relative values are changed infrequently. Necessary adjustments to the specifications of this schedule are advised by a three-party committee. The monetary multipliers are re-negotiated annually between the sickness funds and unions of independent doctors, who try to reach national agreements ('convention nationale') on contracts and conditions. Individual doctors have the freedom to quit the convention (to be 'non conventionné'). In fact almost all doctors join the convention.

Those who subscribe to the convention can be divided into two groups. The largest group (75%) bills according to the fee schedule, and their patients are reimbursed the full charge minus the co-payment rate. A second group consists of doctors designated by the sickness fund because of their academic position, experience or professional reputation. These doctors may charge higher fees (les dépassements). The patient, however, must pay the surplus amount. A third, very small group, only two percent of the doctors, does not conform to the convention and is free to fix fees themselves. Their patients are reimbursed at a very low rate.

The sickness funds have little or no control over the volume of medical services or the location of the doctors. However, they do monitor the volume of each doctor's activity and feed back the results in the hope that this will influence the volume of activity. Excessive prescribing may be sanctioned.

General practitioners in health centres and hospital-based physicians are salaried.

Public hospitals and private non-profit hospitals taking part in the public hospital service have had global, prospective budgets for operating expenses since 1984. These are shared by the local statutory insurers in proportion to the number of bed-days consumed in their catchment are. The budgets include depreciation and interest on capital and are based on historical levels of expenditure. A rate of increase for all global budgets is set centrally, with little scope for local deviation. The budgets are divided into 12 monthly allocations and distributed to the hospital through a local sickness fund referred to as the "caisse pivot".

Most private hospitals are reimbursed on a per diem basis for in-patient care, with separate fee-for-service payments for physician services under the same convention, which applies to ambulatory care. The rates cover depreciation and interest on capital. They are negotiated between the hospitals and the statutory insurers under government guidelines about the permitted annual rate of price increases.

The statutory health insurance system also plays an important part in financing long-term care, much of which is provided by the hospital system.

6.6 *Policy developments in health care*

As in other countries cost containment is the most important issue in health care policy in France. In this respect the introduction of global hospital budgets is considered to be successful. Government policy is more oriented towards a sectoral evaluation of health care than towards the definition of an overall health policy. It continues to improve the performance of the health care system by a succession of more modest reforms. The Hospital Law (1991) centred on three major issues:

- a desire to implement regional planning for the whole of the hospital system (public and private) thus improving the "health care map";
- a need to strengthen the autonomy of the public hospital system;
- a wish to standardise regulations relating to establishments in the public and private sector.

Measures proposed to reduce expenses have included the imposition of limits on medical fees and the removal of refunds for a growing list of non-essential pharmaceuticals.

An experimental new form of regulation, based on "target contracts" which determine a maximum increase in expenditure at national and regional level for 1992, has been agreed between the government, the social security system and certain health care professionals. This has already been implemented for ambulance drivers, nurses, biologists and private clinics. Under the proposals, patients would register with a single family doctor and enjoy third party payment and an annual health statement. The doctor would receive a fixed amount from the sickness fund for each person on his list and the annual health statement would be used for epidemiological studies. In hospitals an attempt has been made to adapt the concept of diagnosis related groups (DRG's) to the French health care system.

The development of medical information systems in both intramural and extramural care is envisaged in order to increase knowledge about medical activities per pathology.

6.7 *Organisation of health care*

6.7.1 *General characteristics*

The French health care system is sometimes characterized as a reconciliation of solidarity and liberalism by means of a combination of collective financing and a public and private sector for the delivery of care. On the one hand there are the social principles embodied in the national health insurance schemes, and on the other liberal principles resulting in the independent medical practice (la médecine libérale) and the large freedom of choice for patients. There is strong government influence in the intramural sector. Extramural care is predominantly operated privately.

Patients are free to choose the medical doctor they want, whether he/she is a general practitioner or a specialist in his/her own cabinet, or a specialist at a hospital. Also in the case of hospital admission patients are free to choose the hospital. The general practitioner does not function as a "gatekeeper", and patients are not registered with a doctor. It is sometimes even attractive for patients to visit hospitals immediately, if costs for the care needed are almost entirely reimbursed. However, generally speaking, co-payments (ticket modérateur) seem to be the only instrument to regulate patient flows.

6.7.2. *Intramural care*

Hospitals in France can be classified in several ways. A basic division takes length of stay as criterion: short stay, medium stay and long stay hospitals. According to Schneider et al. this classification has only statistical significance, as acute hospitals (short stay services) also have departments for medium and long stay. The distinction between public and private hospitals is more important. For public hospitals there is a kind of hierarchy:

- regional hospital centres in the greater health regions; these regional hospitals are also teaching hospitals and therefore equipped with all specialisms and with research facilities.
- hospital centres, which are general hospitals or specialised hospitals (other than psychiatric hospitals), established to cope with the basic health needs of the community. These hospitals have all basic specialisms of medicine, surgery and maternity care, but no "top-specialisms".
- local hospitals, providing general medicine and care for the elderly. They have no emergency department. The care for the elderly is an important feature of hospitals in France. According to Van der Werff French public hospitals contain about 120,000 beds for the elderly.

Private hospitals can be divided into non-profit hospitals and for-profit hospitals. Many non-profit, private hospitals take part in the public hospital service and are financed under the same budget system as public hospitals. Other private hospitals are paid at day prices with separate fee-for-service payments for physician services. For their investments they depend on loans from banks and other private sources like philanthropic grants.

Public hospitals tend to be large, well equipped and under duty to deal with accidents and emergencies. They have limited dispensation to treat private patients. Private hospitals are smaller and specialise in elective surgery, obstetrics or medium and long term care. Most hospitals have outpatient departments. Patients are free to choose between public or private hospitals. The difference in the payment system has no consequences for patients.

The planning of hospitals is operated at regional level with the "carte sanitaire" as planning instrument. Military hospitals and prison hospitals are included in hospital statistics.

6.7.3 *Extramural care*

Extramural care is predominantly privately operated. Patients are free to choose the medical doctor they want, whether he/she is a general practitioner or a specialist in his/her own cabinet, or a specialist at a hospital. Also in the case of hospital admission patients are free to choose the hospital. Thermal cures and laboratory tests outside hospitals are also included under this category of care.

6.7.3.1 *Medical care*

Extramural health care is provided both by general practitioners and independent specialists working from their own premises. Also many hospital specialists have private practices.

The general practitioner does not function as a "gatekeeper", and patients are not registered with a doctor. In most cases the general practitioner is an independent doctor, practising alone. A small number work in health centres, which are established by municipalities, voluntary societies and other organisations like local health insurance funds and labour unions. These health centres are generally recognised as part of the social security system.

6.7.3.2 *Dental care*

Most dentists work as self-employed entrepreneurs, but dental assistance may also be sought in health centres and hospitals.

6.7.3.3 *Pharmacists*

Pharmacists are also self-employed entrepreneurs, but subject to many government regulations.

6.7.3.4 *Paramedical care*

Extramural care is completed by the care of physiotherapists, orthoptists speech therapists, dieticians and psychologists. However, psychologists are not counted as health care professionals.

6.7.3.5 Home nursing and home care

With regard to home care a distinction is made between home care of a medical kind (home nursing) and home care of a social kind (home help, meals-on wheels etc.). Only the medical kind is paid for by the sickness funds and, by consequence, included in the health accounts.

Two organisations are active in the field of home nursing: SIAD (Soins infirmiers à domicile pour personnes âgées) and HAD (Hospitalisation à domicile).

HAD-service can be viewed as a substitute for complete or partial hospitalisation with comparable nursing care. SIAD provides continuous, lighter care, especially for the elderly.

In addition to these organisations with salaried workers, there are a large number of self-employed nurses, the "libérales". They can be hired by a patient, but also by home nursing organisations. In order to control the development of the "libérales" the government has set limits, beyond which activities are no longer remunerated.

6.7.3.6 Extramural mental health care services

Psychiatric care has shown a strong decrease of complete hospitalisation in favour of other modalities of care: partial hospitalisation or ambulatory care. In 1981 60% of adult patients in general psychiatry were admitted to complete intramural care, compared with 13% in 1993. Ambulatory mental care is provided by the Centres Psychiatriques d'Orientation et d'Accueil, the consultation units of the Centres médico-psychologiques or by physicians and their assistants visiting their patients at home or in the homes for the elderly.

Ambulatory mental health care is provided also by psychiatric specialists, practising from their own premises or connected to private clinics, or by psychologists and psychoanalysts, not being psychiatrists.

In the health accounts only the costs of self employed physicians are presented under the entry "soins ambulatoires".

6.7.3.7 Extramural centres for alcohol and drugs addicts

"Centres d'hygiène alimentaire et d'alcoologie" exist since 1970. In 1987 there were 247 of these centres. They are easy accessible for the intake of patients, but also for crisis intervention and therefore open permanently. They are places for the treatment and re-education of excessive drinkers. Personnel are composed of physicians and social workers. Another task of these centres is prevention, especially by intervention at the working place and in schools, universities and hospitals.

Treatment of alcohol patients is provided also by self employed physicians, generalists as well as specialists.

Centres specialised in the care of drug addicts are predominantly financed by the central government. Drug addicts, treated in these centres don't pay for their treatment or aftercare, but only for their protected shelter, if they are lodged with the perspective of re-integration. The centres must fulfil at least the following functions:

- medical and psychological treatment of the addict;
- social care and education, directed to integration or re-integration;
- relief and information for the drug addicts and their families;
- withdrawal and its guidance, until realised in a hospital environment;
- support of the family of the addict.

The centres also can participate in preventive activities and in training and research in the field of drug addiction. They can be managed by private, non-profit organisations or by public health institutions. They also can be governed directly by State services.

Therapeutic dwellings exist since 1993: In this system, adult addicts are treated by a medical staff and live in an independent way with the aim to re-integrate, not realisable in a collective lodging system. In the same perspective drug addicts can be placed in host families, under the responsibility of the addiction centre and under continued treatment.

6.7.3.8 Ambulance services and patient transport

The term transport of patients in France relates to the transport of patients (the sick, injured, pregnancies) by means of a form of transport specially equipped for that purpose, by land sea or air, in connection with medical care or diagnostics, by medical prescription or in event of emergency.

There are 4 categories of land transport:

- 'ambulance de secours et soins d'urgence' (ambulances, equipped for rendering first aid and special care in emergency situations)
- 'voiture de secours d'urgence aux asphyxiés et blessés (VSAB) ' (ambulances, equipped for rendering first aid and transporting the injured and others in having difficulty in breathing)
- ambulance (standard ambulance)
- 'véhicule sanitaire léger' (vehicle for transporting patients who are only slightly ill/injured)

The companies involved require the approval of the prefect of the relevant department. The Ministry of Health is responsible for setting down the standards for the categories A, C and D.

The Ministry of Home Affairs is the authority for category B, the VSAB's, which falls under the fire brigade.

In France there is an organisational difference between the transporting of patients in vehicles with and without a doctor on board.

Transport without a doctor is executed by a private enterprise, or by the fire brigade VSAB's. The private enterprise acts solely as directed on medical prescription.

The (voluntary) fire brigade not only comes into action to fight fires, but also in cases of accidents on public roads. The fire brigade renders first aid to the injured and provides the necessary transport.

Ambulance staff, both drivers and other staff, have all had special training. The same applies for the ambulance personnel of the fire brigade.

The medical ambulance transport (with doctor on board) is done by the "Services mobiles d'urgence et de réanimation" (SMUR) or by certain fire brigade ambulances. A SMUR team is made up of at least one driver-stretcher-bearer, nurse and a doctor, qualified in treating road-accident victims and resuscitation. A SMUR ambulance has special apparatus and medicine on board for resuscitation and patient care (monitoring). The SMUR must have a permit from the Ministry of Health, that supervises compliance of the regulations.

At hospitals with a regional function for receiving accident victims, there are landing areas for helicopters close by the first aid station.

The sickness funds and medical insurance companies pay for cost relating to the transport of patients, even when the transport is done by a private car, taxi or train.

6.7.3.9 Medical laboratories

Medical laboratories outside hospitals are private laboratories. They numbered 4100 in 1995. Since 1988 anatomo-cyto-pathology can be exercised by self employed physicians practising this specialism from their own premises. Since then the medical laboratories are no longer the only to practice this specialism.

6.8 *Preventive health care*

Apart from preventive care intertwined with curative care preventive care services have been developed at individual and collective level. At individual level GP's, Mother & Child Protection centres and the Dispensaries ("dispensaires") play an important role. The "dispensaires" may be polyvalent or specialised: vaccination, TBC-abatement, sexually transmitted diseases, AIDS, family planning, food hygiene, abuse of alcohol, drugs and tobacco, sports medicine.

At the level of collective prevention there are services for school health and industrial health. In the field of health protection services have been organised at national, departmental and municipal level. Their activities are especially directed to public hygiene, e.g. the surveillance of foodstuffs, drinking water and environmental hygiene. Distinct services have been created for the prevention of industrial accidents.

6.9 *Medical goods*

Medical goods include two categories: the category of pharmaceuticals and the category of therapeutic appliances.

6.9.1 *Pharmaceuticals*

Pharmaceutical consumption is high. In order to control the costs of this a positive list has been introduced. The Medicines Directorate must approve pharmaceuticals for reimbursement. If a drug offers no therapeutic advantages over its rivals, it is only listed if its price is lower. With regard to pharmaceuticals there are differences as to the urgency. For patients suffering from chronic diseases, as listed on an official list of about 30 severe pathologies, drugs, prescribed with regard to these diseases, are reimbursed completely.

Other drugs require co-payments of 35 or 65% or even 100%.

6.9.2 *Therapeutic appliances*

In France a large package of therapeutic appliances is included in the health accounts. Only wigs and elastic stocking are completely excluded.

6.10 *Other services*

Other services consist of activities, that in general are not be defined as health care in a strict sense, but of activities, of which the costs are adopted in the national health accounts of many countries.

In France the education of health care personnel is included in the health account as is the health care research. The expenditures of the health insurance funds are excluded from the expenditures in the administrative area. The expenditures of private insurance companies in the area of health insurance are partially included in the health accounts.

7. Country profile: Switzerland

7.1 Introduction

The exchange of information in the network of experts facilitated the production of the "country profiles", which are meant to provide:

- a quick introduction to the organisation and administration of the health care systems of the participating countries
- an exploration of the boundaries of the health care systems
- a preliminary determination of place and functions of health care
- an overview of the main policy developments
- a contribution to transparency, a necessary condition for international comparison.

The country profiles contain information on health care administration, financing, policy developments and the organisation of health care. This information was brought together in the two phases of the project "international comparison of health care data".

In the first phase (1994–1995) the boundaries of the national health care systems were explored. Also general characteristics of health care administration, financing, policy developments and health care organisation were described.

Detailed quantitative data became available on intramural health care. The expression "intramural health care" proved to be a typically Dutch one. Intramural health care is by and large equal to in-patient health care or stationary care. The description used (see Annex 2.4) is health care for patients formally admitted for a period of more than 24 hours and/or institutionalised treatment for a substantial part of the day (or night).

In the second phase of the project (1996–1997) more detailed data were collected on extramural care, preventive health care, medical goods and other services. Also attention was paid to an update of the determination of the boundaries of national health care systems.

Also the expression "extramural health care" proved to be a typically Dutch one. Extramural health care is described as health care provided on a non-residential basis by medical and paramedical professionals or by specialised organisations in home care or home nursing (for a complete description see Annex 2.4).

At the start of the project the intention was to provide country profiles for all the sectors of care described in this report. This goal was not reached. Especially

information on the topic of "other services" is lacking. To a lesser extent the same holds true for the topic of "medical goods".

Dr. M. Wyss, from the Federal Office of Statistics (FOS) Bern, produced the country profile of Switzerland.

7.2 *Aspects of general administration of health care*

In the political context Switzerland is a federal state comprising 26 cantons (States). The Federal Assembly is composed of two assemblies: the National Council (220 members) and the Council of States (46 members). The federal government has 7 members elected by the Federal Assembly; one of the seven is elected President of the Swiss Confederation each year and for one year. The main political power is in the hands of the people. Any change in the Swiss Constitution has to be accepted by the Swiss people (mandatory referendum). By the rights of optional referenda and initiatives, almost any issue may be submitted to popular vote.

The health system is to be understood in this political context. The Swiss health system is organized on a decentralized and federal basis in which the private sector is predominant. An important principle of the Swiss Federal Constitution, the right of self-regulation in the free economy, the "Handels- und Gewerbefreiheit", is also effective and powerful in the Swiss health care system. At the levels of the states, which composes the Federal State, it is also essentially the cantons, which determine the number and the level of the services of their own public health systems.

In Switzerland, there is no Ministry of Health at federal level. The Federal Office of Public Health (BAG) and the Federal Office for Social Insurance (BSV) have at federal level only a few tasks in response to the Swiss federal constitution:

- National health promotion/prevention policies and strategies concerning AIDS, illegal drugs, alcohol and tobacco);
- Surveillance of infectious diseases;
- Surveillance of radioactivity;
- Food Control ;
- Surveillance of medical degrees (Federal Law and reglements of examination in medicine);
- National accident insurance (UVG);
- National old age and disability insurance (AHV/IV).
- Surveillance of social sickness funds.

Both of the offices are part of the Federal Department (Ministry) of the Interior. The main responsibilities are at state level especially health care.

The Conference of Cantonal Directors for Health Affairs (SDK), which acts as an intercantonal co-ordinator, deals, among others with problems relating to the planning and management of the health system, which are common to all the cantons. Another intercantonal office (IKS) is regulating the drug market. The decentralised, federal structure of the Swiss health system, alongside the wide range of tasks and competencies, explain why there is no single body responsible for health service provision and planning. Especially in ambulatory care, the private sector plays an overriding role, without however observing purely market economy rule due to social insurance laws. It can be said Switzerland has a "paradox of ungovernability and efficacy" in relation to the Swiss health system.

7.3 *Financing of health care*

For the year 1991 the social security system is the main source with nearly half of total contributions (49,7%), although the households (29%), the State (19%) (Confederation, cantons and municipalities) and residents of other countries (2,3%) contribute to the other half of the burden.

7.4 *Insurance structure*

The system of social sickness insurance in Switzerland is a part of the system of social security and has been regulated by federal law (Kranken-und Unfallversicherungs-gesetz, KUVG) since 1911 revised 1964). In general the coverage is individual, although 3 cantons declared insurance compulsory. Almost 100% of the population is insured in accordance with this not really obligatory system. The social sickness insurance is now (1992) operated by 191 sickness funds, which are co-ordinated by the Federation of health insurance companies (Konkordat der schweizerischen Krankenkassen, KSK). This umbrella organisation has a statistical function of co-ordination between the sickness funds and the Confederation or the cantons. These funds are required to operate on a non-profit principle, to provide equal treatment to all insured persons, to provide at least the minimum standard benefits and adequate financial security to meet their needs and to accept periodic audits by the Federal Office for Social Insurance. Funding is primarily by contributions of insured persons. All insured have to pay 10 percent as retain for ambulatory treatments, but there is no co-payment for hospitalisation costs. There is also a fixed annual franchise fee (min. SFr. 150,-) Additionally, there are also private insurance companies offering sickness insurance schemes.

The accident insurance provides compulsory coverage for all employed persons. Self-employed are included on a voluntary basis at the same rates. The scheme is administered by the Swiss National Accident Insurance Institute (SUVA) or through private insurance companies which had a market share of about 30% in 1992.

7.4.1 *Sickness funds benefits*

The statutory sickness insurance scheme in Switzerland covers in an individual way (at a basis of a private contract) an extensive package of benefits: ambulatory care by medical doctors, ambulatory treatments by paramedical professionals (physiotherapists, chiropractitioner, etc.), after referral by a physician, pharmaceuticals, intramural care up to 720 consecutive days and rehabilitation services. Special features of the sickness fund benefits in Switzerland are co-payments of treatment costs at a health spa (Kurort).

However, general dental care, preventive examinations and home care (nursing, home help) are not included.

7.4.2 *Cost sharing*

Hospitals and to a lesser extent the nursing homes and the home care are subsidised by the cantonal authorities.
The national disability insurance is financed by the Confederation (50%), employers (25%) and employees (25%). The accident insurance is financed by employers for the occupational risks and by employees for non-occupational risks.

Since the mid 1970s, diminishing public subsidies and rising health costs have put an increasing burden on households, particularly for the low and middle income classes (groups).
By direct payments (29%) or by payments to sickness funds (32,4%), the households contribute to 61 % of the total health care costs.

The participation of the various payers varies considerably, depending on the type of service in question: the public authorities are financing a considerable percentage of the costs of hospitals (cantons) and home care (municipalities and cantons). In contrast, there is no public sector contribution to outpatient medical care, 79% of expenditure being covered by social insurance and 21% by the patients themselves including reimbursement from private insurance companies. 94% of dental care costs are directly defrayed by the patients (BFS, 1994).

7.5 *Fee and salary structure*

Medical doctors in private practice are billing their services on a fee for service basis regulated by contracts between their own association and the cantonal sickness funds. Medical doctors working in hospitals are paid by salary. Day rates for treatments of non-private patients are fixed between hospital associations and sickness funds in each of the 26 cantons. The Federation of health insurance companies (Konkordat der schweizerischen Krankenkassen, KSK) publishes a complete list of hospital tariffs called "Day prices in hospitals" (Tagestaxen in Heilanstalten) twice a year.

In case of conflicts between hospitals, sickness funds and Cantons, the Confederation decides on the basis of the costs of comparable hospitals and regional economic indicators. Additionally, treatment costs for private patients are billed on a fee for service basis. Insured patients are reimbursed by sickness funds for bills concerning ambulatory care services. In general the hospital bills are paid directly by the sickness funds.

7.6 *Policy developments in health care*

The steady growth of the elderly population as well as the continuing rise in unemployment and poverty will generate an even higher demand on medical services. The Swiss population is unlikely to accept a reduced provision of services and a lower quality of care. Rationing access to care will remain highly unpopular.

The shortage of nurses of Swiss nationality is likely to grow. In the course of the process of European integration, the number of foreign nurses working in Switzerland is expected to decline. Domestic recruitment efforts will have to be accompanied by wage increases and improved working conditions to compete with professions such as teaching and social work.

The number of physicians will continue to increase, even if access to medical schools is restricted by the possible introduction of a numerus clausus. A few cantons are attempting to contain hospitalisation costs by means of fixed annual budgetary allocations. While hospital administrators are under pressure to reduce the length of stay, cantons and local communities are starting to set up alternative structures to avoid unnecessary hospitalisation. Although federal authorities lack the formal competence to adopt a national "Health for All"(HFA)-strategy, HFA principles are increasingly being taken into account at cantonal level. National health promotion/ prevention policies and strategies have been established by the Federal Office for Public Health (AIDS, drugs, alcohol and tobacco) and the Swiss Foundation for Health Promotion (health at the work place, adolescent health and cancer prevention).

Debates over the last decade have focused on the financial situation of the health insurance companies. There is widespread agreement that the practice of selecting 'good risks' must be stopped in order to maintain social solidarity. Despite widespread opposition, the federal government recently decided on several urgent measures: compulsory risk compensation payments among insurance companies, a maximum premium increase of 10% per annum and a symbolic patient participation of about sFr. 10.- per day of hospitalisation.

Since 1990, new health insurance schemes have been in evaluation, especially Health Maintenance Organisations (HMO) and the bonus-system (consumption based premium).

7.7 *Organisation of health care*

7.7.1 *General characteristics*

An important characteristic of the Swiss health system is the division between ambulatory care and hospital care. In general, hospitals do not offer outpatient care but they do it more and more often, for instance for and after surgery. In general, doctors working in extramural care do not have access to hospital facilities, but this depends on the "medical care system" of the hospital. There are doctors employed in hospitals who are treating outpatients in addition on a private basis or "Belegärzte" / "médecins agréés" who manage the intramural care in a private way. More than 90 % of the doctors are member of the Swiss Medical Association (FMH) which regulates specialist training and continuous medical education. Working permissions for private doctors are given by the cantonal governments.

In 1991, the Swiss health system currently employs over 350 000 persons, i.e. 9,3% of the entire working population of the country. This figure not only includes doctors, nursing and paramedical staff, but also the personnel of socio-medical institutions (e.g. special schools, rehabilitation centres) and administrative and back-up services (e.g. hospitals, health insurance).

In 1990, Switzerland had a total of 21462 physicians, 4357 dentists, 8116 physiotherapists; a total of 193762 health professionals was active in the field of intramural and extramural care (census data FOS).

The majority of hospitals and non-hospital health care institutions in Switzerland (a total of 2759 establishments) are institutions under public law or under public control receiving substantial subsidies from the public authorities).

Patients are free to choose their doctor. This can be a general practitioner or a specialist. For hospital admission the patient needs a referral by an ambulatory care doctor (excluding emergency cases or direct referrals from the hospitals outpatient department).

Sickness fund patients normally are referred to the nearest hospital with suitable facilities. Private patients and sickness fund patients having either additional insurance coverage for private treatment or having special treatment needs, can be referred to hospitals outside the area of residence.

7.7.2 *Intramural care*

In 1991, 308 of the 398 hospitals are acute care hospitals (physical illness), 90 are psychiatric clinics. The acute care admission rate is 14,9 per 100 inhabitants, in 1992. More than 1 million cases of hospitalisation are recorded annually in Switzerland.

Among this category 229 hospitals including university hospitals are general hospitals, 79 are specialised clinics. Highly specialised health services are provided by the university hospitals of Zurich, Basle, Bern, Lausanne and Geneva.
Acute hospitals are distinguished from long term chronic care institutions. The total number of hospital beds is 57468: 45159 for acute care, 12309 in psychiatric care.

The occupancy rate is 79% for hospitals providing short-term treatment, 83% for psychiatric clinics. The average length of stay in hospitals providing short-term treatment is 13 days, 126 days in psychiatric clinics. The average length of hospitalisation in acute care has fallen from 26 to 13 days over the last three decades. In 1991, Swiss hospitals employed a total of some 105000 persons (full-time equivalents): 91000 in short-term establishments, 14000 in psychiatric clinics.

Long term care is given in geriatric clinics and in non-hospital health care institutions. In 1991, there were 10 geriatric clinics with 1458 beds. The occupancy rate is 92% for geriatric clinics. The average length of stay in geriatric clinics is 55 days.

Non-hospital health care establishments include homes of the elderly (irrespective of their degree of medical or nursing care), institutions for the disabled, drug addicts or alcoholics. Also thermal baths, spa, convalescent, dietic, climatic, preventative and psycho-social treatment centres (including post cure) (Federal Office of Statistics, 1992). Nursing homes and homes for the elderly are run by local authorities and voluntary bodies. They are financed mainly by private expenditure, often supported by public assistance. The national insurance for the elderly, survivors and disabled (AHV, IV) provide benefits in case of income or fortune insufficiency (Ergänzungsleistungen).

- The 2351 so-called non-hospital establishments offer 125874 beds or places, whereas all institutions for the elderly (nursing homes, medico-social institutions, etc.) and the institutions for the disabled provide 111956 (89%) of the total number of beds or places available in this sector.
- In 1991, more than 89000 persons (or 64077 full-time equivalents) were employed by the non-hospital establishments. The majority of the workforce provides care (39%). Caterers (25%), social workers (21%), specialised therapeutic personnel (4%), doctors (1%) and administrative, technical and annex staff (11%) account for a much smaller proportion. In general the occupancy rate is 96%.

7.7.3 Extramural care

7.7.3.1 Medical care

Extramural care is mainly provided by independent general practitioners and specialists. Other health professionals are often involved as employees of physicians.

Patients are free to choose their doctor. This can be a general practitioner or a specialist. For hospital admission the patient needs a referral by an ambulatory care doctor (excluding emergency cases or direct referrals from the hospitals outpatient department). Ambulatory practices are well equipped and have ample access to most diagnostic services. There is a predominance of independent doctors in single practices, although partnerships, usually of two doctors in the same speciality are growing in number. Common use of diagnostic equipment and laboratory facilities are the advantages of these types of co-operation. In general, doctors working in extramural care do not have access to hospital facilities, but this depends on the "medical care system" of the hospital. There are doctors employed in hospitals who are treating out-patients in addition on a private basis or "Belegärzte"/"médecins agréés" who manage the intramural care in a private way. Medical doctors are organised in the Swiss Medical Association (Federatio Medicorum Helveticorum), which regulates specialist training and continuous medical education. These medical professionals are partners with the cantonal institutions and the cantonal health insurance funds, which are organised in the Federation of health insurance funds (Konkordat der schweizerischen Krankenkassen, KSK).
There are free contracts between the health insurance funds and the doctor's association's institutions in every canton. In case of conflicts, first the cantonal government and after that the federal government can decide. This is also true for hospital prices. Working permissions for private doctors are given by the cantonal governments. In 1992, Switzerland had a total of 11120 physicians in private practice, 4030 of whom or 36% are general practitioners and 64% specialised physicians (FMH). The number of specialists varies considerably from canton to canton and is higher in cantons with a higher degree of urbanisation.
Medical surgeries provide some 75 million consultations per year. This means that each inhabitant consults a doctor on average eleven times a year as an outpatient (FMH 1992). Physicians in private practice carry out 95% of out-patient medical consultations (Hausser et al. 1990); the remaining 5% take place in hospitals.

7.7.3.2 Dental care

Patients are free to choose their dentist. Dentists are organised in the "Schweizerische Zahnärzte-Gesellschaft" (SS0). There are no fee contracts between the sickness funds, but with accident insurance (national scheme), and the organisation of the dentists (SSO). Patients are own payers, except in case of accident. There were 3368 dentists in private practice in 1992 or 2060 inhabitants per one practice. This corresponds to 73 percent of all dentists (Census data 1990).

7.7.3.3 Pharmacists

Pharmacists are organised in the "Schweizerischer Apothekerverein". There were 1562 pharmacies in 1992 or one pharmacy for 4444 inhabitants. This is equivalent to 1157 pharmacists or 34 percent of all pharmacists (Census data in 1990).

In 1994, the drug market in Switzerland amounted to 3.7 billion CHF (Pharma Information, Basel 1995). This corresponds to more than 10 percent of the total health care expenditures. From this total amount, 62 percent are delivered in pharmacies, 19 percent by medical doctors (Selbstdispensation), 12 percent in hospitals and 7 percent in druggist's shops. 64 percent of medicaments for humans are imported and more than a third is produced in Switzerland. More than 90 percent of all medicaments for humans produced in Switzerland are exported. The export amounts to almost 12 billion CHF in 1994. The import/export balance has a surplus of 8 billion CHF (Expertenkommission Heilmittelgesetz (HMG, 1996)".

7.7.3.4 Paramedical care

Professionals in paramedical activities have to follow medical directives based on medical diagnosis and treatment regimen (except for professionals in psychotherapy and in chiropractice who can execute treatment based on their proper diagnosis). Sickness funds pay for paramedical treatments (except for cases not supervised by doctors).

In 1991, there were 3543 practices with about 15 000 employers (professionals) and employees (including professionals and auxiliaries): 879 practices in psychotherapy with 1920 occupied persons, 249 practices in chiropractic with 543 persons, 1382 practices in physiotherapy and ergonomic therapy with 3887 persons, 1033 practices of independent nurses, midwifes etc., with 8117 persons.

7.7.3.5 Home nursing and home care

There exists an unknown number of non-hospital services and care (SPITAL externe Krankenpflege, alias SPITEX): e.g. nursing care at home and family help services, household assistants and meals on wheels, especially for the elderly.

On the basis of a recent survey (Swiss Health Survey, Bern 1994) we know that in 1993, 20 percent of the elderly (85 and older) with handicaps need home care.

Since 1992 home care is a distinct category in the health expenditure statistics. Up to 1991 it was counted among other ambulatory care. About 600 millions are spent for this sector or 2% of the total health expenditures. This sector is increasing.

The estimate is based on the accounts of the National old age and disability insurance (AHV/IV).

7.7.3.6 Extramural mental health care services

No data available.

7.7.3.7 Extramural centres for alcohol and drug addicts

In 1993, there were 184 specialised extramural institutions. A new survey (Statistik der ambulanten Behandlung und Betreuung im Alkohol- und Drogenbereich [SAMBAD]) on a voluntary basis gave indications about the structure of the professionals (professional orientation: most are social workers or psychologists) and the patients (clients: 67 percent are men) and also the kind of consumed drugs (with a predominance of alcohol and heroin).

In the present conception of the health expenditure statistics this field is partly covered in the intramural psychiatric institutions and partly in the occupational and social rehabilitation (disabled persons). That's why a clear cut between intramural institutions and extramural services is problematic and cannot be made. More specific results are not available.

7.7.3.8 Ambulance services and patient transport

The transport of patients in Switzerland is done by ambulance services coupled to hospitals (51%), independent "Rettungsdiensten" of private organisations, with or without profit motive (27%) and municipal services (22%), like the municipal health service or the police.

These services have at their disposal a wide variety of ambulances ("Krankenwagen, Rettungswagen, Notartzwagen") and helicopters.
The costs related to the transport of patients generally falls under the costs of health care. Normally, the emergency ambulance services is an element of the health account.

Financing transport requested for recumbent patients is done through the sickness funds, private health insurance and personal contributions. The sums involved are not known. Normally payment is done indirectly through the sickness funds. There is no compensation for other forms of patient transport (taxis, wheelchair buses, private car), except for persons recognised as handicapped.

7.7.3.9 Medical laboratories

In 1991, there were 157 medical laboratories (Federal Business Survey) with 3073 employees. Data are available all 5 years.

This field is covered by the financial sources (Federal Office for Social Insurance). Financial data are available.

7.8 *Preventive health care*

Up to the early 1980s, the activity of public bodies (Confederation and Cantons) was limited to traditional tasks such as surveillance of food quality, vaccinations, etc.

Health education was carried out by private agencies in the areas of road accident prevention, alcohol, cancer. School health programs are providing immunisations, dental check-ups and tuberculosis screening.

In 1982/83, on the basis of their competence in the area of health, the cantons rejected the introduction of a federal law on health prevention. A number of initiatives have nevertheless been taken at the national level: – In 1983 and 1986, the Swiss Society for Social and Preventive Medicine elaborated a concept "Health Promotion and Prevention in Switzerland" recommending the creation of a prevention unit at the Swiss Office for Public Health (BAG) and the establishment of a special fund for health promotion. Both these recommendations have been followed.

The Swiss Foundation for Health Promotion (Schweizerische Stiftung für Gesundheitsförderung) was created in 1989 by the Cantons, the Confederation, the Swiss association of private insurance companies and the Federation of Sickness Funds (KSK). Despite its very modest budget of some 2,4 million Swiss francs, a number of projects has already been subsidised (prevention in the areas of alcoholism, tobacco dependence, sexual abuse of children, general health education). The Foundation has just issued proposals for a concerted national action in the field of health promotion for the years 1993-97. National priority topics, approved by all relevant public and private institutions are: health at the workplace, adolescent health and cancer prevention.

The Confederation focuses its activities on infectious diseases, Aids, illegal drugs, tobacco and alcohol. In particular, the Confederation has funded the well-known national STOP AIDS campaign since 1987 and another national campaign aiming at the prevention of illegal drugs since 1992. Despite growing awareness of the need for health promotion as well as disease and accident prevention, only very limited resources are earmarked for this area (2% of total health expenses in 1991). Although the role of the family is well-recognised, there is no central strategy, programme or organisation in Switzerland aiming at fostering the health supporting functions of the family. National efforts in the areas of Aids and drug prevention have, however, addressed information booklets to parents in order to encourage discussion of these matters within the family.

7.9 *Medical goods*

Medical goods include two categories: the category of pharmaceuticals and the category of therapeutic appliances.

7.9.1 *Pharmaceuticals*

At the end of 1995, 9124 medicaments were registered by the "Interkantonale Kontrollstelle für Heilmittel" (IKS). 85% are medicaments for humans and 15% for animals. Cantons (Federated States) do not register medicaments (except for one canton).

7.9.2 *Therapeutic appliances*

Dental appliances are supplied by dentist's practices. All other therapeutic appliances are to a certain extent supplied by the Other Ambulatory Services.

7.10 *Other services*

Other services consist of activities that in general are not being defined as health care in a strict sense, but of activities of which the costs are adopted in the national health accounts of many countries.

Only the expenditures in the area of administration are included in the health accounts.

8. Country profile: Belgium

8.1 Introduction

The exchange of information in the network of experts facilitated the production of the "country profiles", which are meant to provide:

- a quick introduction to the organisation and administration of the health care systems of the participating countries
- an exploration of the boundaries of the health care systems
- a preliminary determination of place and functions of health care
- an overview of the main policy developments
- a contribution to transparency, a necessary condition for international comparison.

The country profiles contain information on health care administration, financing, policy developments and the organisation of health care. This information was brought together in the two phases of the project "international comparison of health care data".

In the first phase (1994–1995) the boundaries of the national health care systems were explored. Also general characteristics of health care administration, financing, policy developments and health care organisation were described.

Detailed quantitative data became available on intramural health care. The expression "intramural health care" proved to be a typically Dutch one. Intramural health care is by and large equal to in-patient health care or stationary care. The description used (see Annex 2.4) is health care for patients formally admitted for a period of more than 24 hours and/or institutionalised treatment for a substantial part of the day (or night).

In the second phase of the project (1996–1997) more detailed data were collected on extramural care, preventive health care, medical goods and other services. Also attention was paid to an update of the determination of the boundaries of national health care systems.

Also the expression "extramural health care" proved to be a typically Dutch one. Extramural health care is described as health care provided on a non-residential basis by medical and paramedical professionals or by specialised organisations in home care or home nursing (for a complete description see Annex 2.4).

At the start of the project the intention was to provide country profiles for all the sectors of care described in this report. This goal was not reached. Especially

information on the topic of "other services" is lacking. To a lesser extent the same holds true for the topic of "medical goods".

8.2 *Aspects of general administration of health care*

In the context of the development of a federal governmental structure in Belgium certain responsibilities for health care have been delegated from federal government to the authorities of the Flemish, French and German Communities. Federal government is responsible for legislation, financing and insurance, hospital programming and hospital quality norms, prices of medicines, the acces to the health professions (legal requirements to exercise the profession) and the practice of health professionals.

Regional, provincial and local authorities take responsibilities in organising prevention, but also ambulatory curative care: outpatient perinatal health care, outpatient mental health care, medical services for schools, medical services for industry and care for the handicapped.

Many private organisations (non-governmental and non-profit) as well as self-employed medical doctors play an important role in the supply of health care services. Private hospitals outnumber public hospitals. Citizens in Belgium enjoy freedom of choice for health care. They can consult general practitioners of their choice or, without interference, they can consult medical specialists or visit hospital outpatient departments. They can even directly request to be admitted to hospital, in which case the hospital doctor decides whether admission is necessary or not.

8.3 *Financing of health care*

Table 8.1
Belgium: Financial sources, 1990 (percentages of total)

	1990
General taxation	32.0
Social security [1]	54.5
Individual payments	13.5
Private insurance	
Total	100.0

Source: Literature 41.
[1] Including voluntary insurance.

Sickness fund premiums are relatively low in Belgium. High government contributions and a large number of co-payments supplement them. Government contributions are used to pay for the health care of the elderly, the disabled, pensioners, widows and orphans.

Investments in hospitals (buildings and expensive equipment) are paid for by the government up to 60 to 100%. Moreover government bears the costs of prevention, like school health care and occupational health care, and some forms of curative care like perinatal care outside hospitals, ambulatory mental care and care for the disabled.

8.4 *Insurance structure*

Health care in Belgium is guaranteed by a system of sickness fund schemes as part of the social security system. Originally only employees and their dependants were covered. By gradual extensions of legislation this system has been made compulsory for almost the whole population (99%). However, rights to be derived from this legislation are different for various groups. Employees and civil servants enjoy complete coverage of risks, but under the compulsory system self-employed people only are insured against high risks like hospitalisation. Persons who do not fall under the compulsory system are offered the possibility to join the social sickness funds voluntarily. The compulsorily insured are obliged to enlist in order to become a member of one of the 129 non-governmental and non-profit sickness funds. There is also freedom of choice with regard to sickness funds. After a certain period the insured can change rather easily from one sickness fund to another.

The sickness funds are grouped into five national associations. Three of them are organised according to the backgrounds of political parties: the National Alliance of Christian Mutual Funds, the National Union of Socialist Mutual Funds and the National League of Liberal Mutualist Federations. Another bears a neutral signature and the last is based on professional backgrounds. Apart from these sickness funds the government has created an assistance fund for sickness and disability (CAAMI). This fund is for those who refuse to join a sickness fund or who neglect to do so.

Due to the almost nation-wide coverage of the social sickness insurance scheme few opportunities are left for private insurance. They have only a supplementary function in the field of minor risks for persons insured under the scheme for the self-employed, in the field of own contributions (extra costs of hospitalisation, drugs etc.) and in the field of expenditures not covered by the sickness funds e.g. certain patient transport costs.
Sickness funds receive their financial resources from the national Office of Social Security, where premiums from employers, employees and self-employed are brought together with governmental subsidies for care for the unemployed, the aged and the poor. INAMI/RIZIV and the national associations of mutualities play a role in the distribution of these resources.

Reimbursement is the leading principle in the social sickness funds insurance in Belgium. This reimbursement is supplied after certification of delivered care. In 1986, however, a "third payer regulation" was introduced creating the possibility of immediate payments by the sickness funds to providers of care. This regulation is obligatory for admission to hospitals and all medical care provided in hospitals.

8.4.1 *Sickness fund benefits*

The law on sickness and disability insurance contains a limitative enumeration of the health care services accepted for reimbursements. This enumeration includes all kinds of preventive and curative care. Four main categories are distinguished: general medical care, specialist care, hospital-nursing care and medicines and medical appliances.

As already indicated benefit packages vary according to employment status. Employees and civil servants are entitled to a broad coverage, including so-called small and high risks. The self-employed are insured against high risks only (e.g. hospitalisation). About 70% of them sign up with a sickness fund or private/profit company for voluntary insurance to cover small risks.

The sickness funds offer their members a broad package of supplementary advantages. Examples are savings schemes before marriage, benefits at marriage and birth, funeral insurance, family help and help for the aged, open air cures and holiday resorts, and recently also legal aid concerning patient rights. For each of these activities a separate bookkeeping is required by law.

8.4.2 *Cost sharing*

Co-payments by patients using health care services are a widespread phenomenon in Belgium. Extramural services must be paid by the patient, and are reimbursed by the sickness fund at a rate of generally 75%. Costs of medicines are reimbursed according to their therapeutic significance. Only four urgent types of medicines are fully reimbursed (antibiotics against TBC and medicines for epileptics and diabetics and chemotherapy for cancer patients). For other medicines co-payments are requested at a rate of 25–75% depending on their therapeutic classification.

In hospitals a fixed amount per day is obliged for boarding costs. Co-payments for physician costs, excluding surgery and gynaecology, are 25%. For the medicines used in hospitals 25 Bfr. have to be paid by the patient.

Specific categories of patients – widows, the disabled, pensioners and orphans – are subject to a less strict scheme.

In the case of industrial accidents and recognised industry-related diseases the patient is entitled to complete reimbursement of payments for medical treatment, medicines and nursing care.

8.5 *Fee and salary structure*

General practitioners and specialists are paid by fee for service. The fee structure is regulated at national level by the National Institute for Sickness and Invalidity Insurance (INAMI/RIZIV). Fees are the results of negotiations between syndicates of medical doctors and sickness funds, followed by negotiations between doctors and hospitals. Agreement between medical doctors and sickness funds must be approved by central government. If no agreement is reached government is entitled by law to fix fees. If an agreement has been reached medical doctors are obliged to bill according to the fee schedule. Some medical doctors, however, do not accept the negotiated fees and in certain circumstances they are free to charge extra. These doctors must announce their non-affiliation to the agreed schedule. Patients making use of their services, are reimbursed according to the agreed fees.

Within the yearly budget of every hospital the Ministry of Health calculates a standard cost price per day, based on historical factors and including more and more so-called production profiles. Factors involved in this calculation are types of medical service, diagnoses, nursing activities and age structure of patients. Other costs are budgetted, taking into account types of medical services, number of beds and age of buildings.

Patients pay a small part of the standard cost price. The Ministry pays 25% of the standard cost price and the remainder is paid by the sickness fund. Medical specialists pay part of their income to the hospital for the use of facilities.

For nursing staff a uniform salary system has been developed for the whole country.

8.6 Policy developments in health care

In recent years several cost containment measures have been introduced in Belgium:

- reimbursement of hospital costs by the Ministry of Health (except medical activities and activities under the RIZIV-nomenclature, reimbursed by the National Institute for Sickness and Invalidity Insu rance, RIZIV/INAMI) will be based on several factors but increasingly on case-mix (pathology grouping of patients), nursing care profiles and specific organisational features of particular services. At present, payment for hospital care is based on a functional budget (main structural characteristics of a hospital) and a supplementary budget (related to the nature and amount of medical and nursing activities, which of course are dependent on the case-mix of a hospital.
- increase of co-payments by patients (especially for drugs) resulting in growing significance of supplementary insurance by sickness funds and private for-profit insurance companies.
- decrease of government subsidies.

- regulation of specific sectors, e.g. prices of medicines and laboratory tests.
- reduction of beds in acute care and psychiatric care in favour of nursing beds for the aged and chronically ill.

In 1990 a new bill on the financing of health care was introduced, of which the main elements are:

- the fixing of a global budget for health care expenditure and several separate budgets for each sector.
- the obligation to implement correction mechanisms when the global or partial budgets are exceeded.
- the creation of a budget control commission entrusted with the supervision of the achievement of budgetary targets and with the task of proposing adjustments to them.
- powers for the Minister to intervene when the care providers and the sickness funds do not succeed in meeting their budgetary targets.

8.7 *Organisation of health care*

8.7.1 General characteristics

The health care system in Belgium is built up of private and public elements: it is mainly privately organised and publicly financed. On the one hand this concerns individual self-employed professionals like general practitioners, specialists, dentists, pharmacists, physiotherapists and others. On the other hand many private non-profit organisations are active in extramural as well as in intramural care. Home nursing is delivered by organisations like the White and Yellow Cross or independent nurses. In the field of intramural care 226 hospitals out of a total of 366 are run by private non-profit organisations in 1993. This dominance is even stronger for psychiatric hospitals, where 58 of a total of 72 hospitals are in private hands. Legislation and public financing offer the general context in which all these elements cooperate.

Given the great freedom of choice indicated above with regard to health care services in Belgium, there is no effective referral system to regulate patient flows. The general practitioner is not the "gatekeeper" of the health care system, as the patient is entitled to visit specialists and hospitals without his interference. Nevertheless for non-medical services referral by medical practitioners is needed: clinical biology, röntgendiagnostics, physiotherapy, nursing care, opticians, acoustic prostheses, bandagist and orthopaedist.

The system of cost-sharing (ticket modérateur) seems to fulfil the function of control on the use of health services more than the referral system.

8.7.2 *Intramural care*

The number of hospitals in Belgium is rather high. Most hospitals (62% in 1993) are in private or semi-private facilities. These are operated by bodies such as sickness funds, religious communities etc. Public hospitals are usually organised by Public Welfare Centres of Municipalities.

Technical control is exercised by the Communities and financial control by the Federal Ministry of Public Health. Hospitals must meet requirements for appropriate structural, architectural, functional and organisational standards and must be compatible with national and regional hospital plans. In 1993 the country counted 366 general hospitals, of which 226 were privately owned and 140 publicly.

Characteristic for both the private and the public sector in Belgium is their small units. In 1985 a policy was adopted aimed at rationalisation by quantitative and qualitative adaptation of the hospital sector. Goals of this policy were the reduction of overall hospital capacity, concentration in hospitals with minimal 150 beds and a well-balanced distribution, taking into account the particular situation of the Brussels Region, where three medical faculties (VUB, ULB, UCL) are established. The results are, that all hospitals have more than 150 beds and that fewer beds are available per 1000 inhabitants.

Since 1986 beds for the chronically ill have been removed from hospitals to Rest and Nursing Homes (Rust- en verzorgingstehuis, RVT). These are no longer considered as hospitals, but constitute necessary links in the range of extramural and intramural facilities for the elderly, of which also geriatric beds in hospitals form a part. The number of beds in general hospitals decreased by 14% in the period 1982–1992. Bed occupancy rates became higher, but the average length of stay in hospitals dropped.

The number of beds in psychiatric hospitals decreased gradually by 27% in the period 1979–1992. In 1990 a reorganisation plan for the psychiatric sector was accepted with less beds, more care facilities and greater collaboration between intra- and extramural care.

8.7.3 *Extramural care*

8.7.3.1 Medical care

Extramural medical care is provided by self-employed general practitioners and specialists. No division of tasks exists between these two categories. The general practitioner is not the "gatekeeper" of the health care system, as the patient is entitled to visit specialists and hospitals without his interference. Nevertheless for specific medical services referral by medical practitioners is needed: clinical biology, radiodiagnostics, physiotherapy, nursing care, opticians, acoustic prostheses, bandagist and orthopaedist.

This, together with a high "doctor density" in Belgium, causes much competition between these categories. General practitioners therefore make many house calls, over 50% of their patient contacts, even if patients are very well capable of coming to the doctor's office. The average number of patient contacts is 11 per day , according to data published by NIVEL in 1993. GPs just starting out have fewer consultations. For younger GPs in particular, sideline jobs are indispensable to make a living.

The solo-practice is the most common form, though there is a change of the attitude among younger general practitioners to join associations (which are mostly still solo's). Group practices occur rarely. For reasons of cost control, Mutualities have created a kind of polyclinics, in which some specialist services are concentrated.

8.7.3.2 Dental care
Dentists are in general self-employed.

8.7.3.3 Pharmacists
Pharmacists are in general self-employed.

8.7.3.4 Paramedical care
Physiotherapists, speech therapists and midwives can either be as independent professionals as well as employees of health care institutions. Within these health care institutions also other paramedical professionals are employed.

8.7.3.5 Home nursing and home care [1)]
There is a strong political tendency to give priority to home care. Generally, home nursing and home help services are separately organised. Only a few organisations provide both kinds of home care. However, in the actual provision of care co-operation between home nurses and home helps is increasing. Home helps sometimes assist home nurses in the daily care of the patient (especially with hygienic tasks) and occasionally signal problems, which they discuss together.

Home nursing services are mainly provided by organisations, which work on a non-profit basis and an increasing number of independent nurses working in private practices. It is estimated that in 1995 about 35% of the market is covered by independent nurses (se literature no. 17).

The largest organisation is the White/Yellow cross which covers the whole country and performs about 50% of all nursing activities. The White/Yellow Cross is divided into three main organisational levels. The actual provision of care is organised at the local level. There are 180 local departments consisting of 20–40 nurses and lead by a head nurse. These departments are controlled and supported by the nine Provincial Cross Associations which determine the number of nurses per region and contract the home nurses. The National Federation of White/Yellow Cross Associations is an umbrella organisation which supports the provincial cross associations, develops policy in co-operation with the provincial cross associations and represents these in contacts with ministries, social associations and professional organisations.

Furthermore there are a number of smaller organisations like Solidariteit voor het Gezin (Solidarity for the Family). This organisation provides both home nursing and home help services, mainly in Eastern Flanders. Its catchment area is divided into nursing regions, which further are divided into sectors in which about 20 nurses and one social nurse are employed. In Walloon an equivalent organisation exists namely the C.D.S. (Centre des Soins à Domicile).

When a person is in need of home nursing, he/she can contact a home nursing organisation or an independent nurse directly. Theoretically, patients have a free choice as to which home nursing organisation they approach, but this choice is often restricted by the limited availability of different organisations in the region. However, recently the opportunity to choose between home care delivered by formal organisations and home care by private nurses has increased enormously. Most patients have a prescription from their physician because a formal authorisation is required for all technical nursing activities such as injections, otherwise the health insurance associations do not reimburse these costs. Only general nursing activities, such as ADL-support, are freely accessible for heavily dependent patients.

After the first contact, a nurse from the home-nursing organisation will visit the patient to assess the patient's level of care dependency. A standardised screening form is used. All nurses who provide home care are also able to fill out the screening forms. Accordingly, the assessment of needs, the actual provision of care and the evaluation of the care provided are mostly the responsibility of the same person. The actual nursing care provided includes hygiene and other personal care, routine technical nursing procedures (injections, stoma care, bladder washouts), more complicated nursing activities (epidural anaesthesia, handling respirator, catheterisation), patient education, and the encouragement of informal care. ADL-assistance, injections and wound dressing are the activities most frequently performed by Belgian home nurses during home visits.

Home nurses from the White/Yellow Cross work in teams co-ordinated by the local departments. In daily practice, most of them operate from their own homes because each nurse takes care of her own specific area.

In general, the organisation of home help services, mainly help with housework, is strictly separated from home nursing activities. Some exceptions are already mentioned, that is Solidariteit voor het Gezin in Eastern Flanders and the Centre des

Soins à Domicile in the Walloon region which provide both home nursing and home help services.

An important distinction must be made between public and private organisations. Although 76% of the home help services organisations are part of the public and 24% to the private sector, the latter accounts for almost 80% of the hours worked.

Each municipality should have its own PCSW, which is in charge of social services in general and services for home help in the family and for the elderly in particular. The municipalities have the authority to control the budget of the centres. There are 589 Public Centres for Social Welfare (PCSW's) in Belgium. These centres own hospitals, old people's homes, and alternative housing units. They organise home help services, cleaning services, job services, service centres and meal distribution. One of the main social functions is to grant the elderly with an insufficient income a benefit equal to the subsistence level and, if necessary, to contribute to the accommodation expenses in the institutions.

The principal professional home help organisations started about 40 years ago, having been based on charity and voluntary work. Private home help organisations are still associated or linked with broader social organisations (e.g. the Christian Workers movement, Socialist movement) and organisations for more specific groups such as the Catholic Pensioners Union, other religious groups, and Health Insurance funds (mutualities). They are also organised at a local level and their catchment area is restricted. Examples of these kinds or organisations are Familiehulp, Familiezorg en Solidariteit voor het Gezin.

Theoretically all clients are free to choose the organisation for home help themselves. However in some regions there are only one or two professional organisations able to provide home help services. No formal referral is needed. So potential clients can contact the home help organisations themselves.

The needs of the potential client are assessed through a so-called social investigation performed by a social worker (or social nurse) who is responsible for the first contact with the client, the work schedule of the home helps and the follow-up.

The next step is the actual provision of home help services by home helps employed by the organisations. All home helps and cleaners operate from their own homes; not from central working units like health centres, hospitals or old people's homes. The work of cleaners is limited to the cleaning of the house. Home helps provide a larger range of care, i.e. housework (preparing meals, washing dishes, washing and ironing, and cleaning), hygienic and other personal care (bathing, ADL-help), moral support (counselling and advice), general and family support (shopping, going for a walk, administrative support), and occasionally encouraging help from family members, neighbours or friends. In practice, the same organisations will provide cleaning as well as home help to the same client.

Home helps provide an average of 11 hours help per week per family, generally the help is spread over two days. The cleaning services deliver help, an average of four hours a week per family. The majority of patients receive help one day per week, but there is a considerable group who only receives cleaning help once in 14 days. This is probably due to the fact that travel costs are not subsidised and therefore need to be kept to a minimum.

8.7.3.6 Extramural mental health care services
No data available

8.7.3.7 Extramural centres for alcohol and drugs addicts
No data available

8.7.3.8 Ambulance services and patient transport
There are 16 emergency centres in Belgium. These are all run with financial support from the Ministries of the Interior and Health. Messages are passed on to the fire brigade, who in turn call the nearest ambulance. These can either belong to a private company, "cross"-organisation (e.g. the Red Cross), the fire brigade itself or a hospital. The ambulance is normally manned with three persons inclusding a nurse. The patient is transported to the nearest hospital. Of the approx. 250 hospitals in Belgium, 180 of these have an emergency service, coupled to an emergency call network. Some hospitals are connected to a "Mobiele Urgentie Groep" or Mobile Urgency Group (MUG), which means that a doctor forms part of the ambulance team.

The emergency services are partially financed through the hospital's daily bed fees. Other ambulance services are dependent on planned transport of patients. The patient pays a rate per kilometre. The compulsory insurance only covers certain cases, for example in the case of serious illnesses, such as with dialysis and cancer patients requiring radiation treatment.

Besides the compulsory insurance, most insurance companies provide supplementary insurance, which includes the coverage of the transport of patients. The extent of coverage differs depending on the insurance. There are no data on how much contribution clients have to pay.

A further item of information with respect to the transport of patients in Belgium, is the existence of the "Minder Mobielen Centrales" (about a hundred in Flanders), who work with volunteers and are partially financed by local authorities. The patients pay a rate per kilometre. This service is normally called in, for instance, to transport patients from and to a hospital or rehabilitation centre. Data on this service are not available.

8.7.3.9 *Medical labatories*

No data available

8.8 *Preventive health care in Belgium*

Preventive health care services are generally organised and financed by public authorities (Communities, provincial and local government, sickness funds), but also private non-profit organisations fulfil tasks in this field. Important areas of activities are outpatient perinatal care, outpatient mental health, medical services for schools, medical services for industry, sport medicine and care for the handicapped. A parastatal organisation, called "Kind en Gezin" (Child and Family), is specialised in preventive health care for children under the age of five years.
In the field of health protection and environmental health the regions, provinces and the "Institute for Hygiene and Environmental Health" play important roles.

8.9 *Medical goods*

Medical goods include two categories: the category of pharmaceuticals and the category of therapeutic appliances.

8.9.1 *Pharmaceuticals*

Costs of medicines are reimbursed according to their therapeutic significance. Only four urgent types of medicines are fully reimbursed (antibiotics against TBC and medicines for epileptics and diabetics and chemotherapy for cancer patients). For other medicines co-payments are requested at a rate of 25–75% depending on their therapeutic classification.

8.9.2 *Therapeutic appliances*

In Belgium all therapeutic appliances are accounted for in the health accounts. However the out of pocket expenditures are not included.

8.10 *Other services*

Other services consist of activities that in general are not being defined as health care in a strict sense, but of activities of which the costs are adopted in the national health accounts of many countries.
In Belgium the income compensation and specific financial support in case of illness or disability is part of the health accounts. Health research expenditures are only partially included. All administrative expenditures are part of the health accounts in Belgium.

Note

1) This paragraph is derived from literature no. 23.

9. *Bilateral Comparisons: framework*

9.1 *Introduction*

This chapter presents the composition process of the Bilateral Comparisons in the health care sector of the participating countries and the general framework which puts the participant's health care sector in an economic context. In this next chapters (chapter 10 through 13) the Bilateral Comparisons on Intramural health care, Extramural health care, Preventive health care and Medical goods will be presented. In chapter 14, the attempted construction of Bilateral Packages on Research & Development and Education & Training is presented. The description of the construction of the Common Comparable Package (CCP) is presented in chapters 16 through 20.

9.2 *Description of the process of bilateral comparison*

Based on the country profiles and on the health care literature a general analysis of functions of health care has been carried out, resulting in a list of health care activities. This list was used to determine activities of distinct health care provisions present in the participating countries.

Next Statistics Netherlands developed a list of provisions available in most of the participating countries. This list of provisions was linked to a questionnaire on the boundaries of care and the cost structure in countries.

The chosen procedure led to matrices on the provisions by cost structure returned by the participants (the constructed Health Accounts). Most of these were accompanied by a lot of annotations. These matrices formed the basic material for the bilateral comparisons.

First all the information on the cost structure was analysed and harmonised as far as possible. Decisions had to be taken on provisions listed as non-existent, and listed as partially in health care. If provisions were listed as non existent, the activities of these provisions might be non-existent as well. The majority of these activities were part of the service package of other health care services.

Partial could mean partially included in the health care system but also partly accounted for in the cost data of health care. Together with the information already present in the country profiles and the list of activities, for every country pair it was possible to create an extensive annotated dataset in local currency units. A country pair always consisted of the Netherlands and one of the other participating countries.

For every bilateral dataset a division was made into a part on comparable data, containing provisions and activities present in both countries (meaning the Netherlands and one other country), and another part containing the provisions not present or not counted as health care provision in the Netherlands and provisions not known or considered as health care in the other country.

Bilateral datasets in local currency units are not easily compared. So a set of common units of measurement and some common denominators were needed, in short some framework data. The OECD Health Data Bank (1997) was chosen for this purpose. The OECD supplies data on dollar exchange rates, Purchasing Power Parities (PPP's), population and Gross Domestic Product (GDP) and data on ECU rates. These framework data facilitated the composition of lists in dollars and ECU's in addition to the lists of provisions in local currency.

9.3 *General framework*

9.3.1 Introduction

The approach taken by Statistics Netherlands was to create a bilateral or country by country comparison. The most important sources of data used for these comparisons are the lists of activities supplied by the different countries and the information concerning services counted in health care and the amounts (in national currency) allocated to these services.

Based on available data five comparisons were made:

- The Netherland – Denmark
- The Netherland – Germany
- The Netherland – France
- The Netherland – Switzerland
- The Netherland – Belgium

In the process of comparing the information on services, health care was divided into blocks:

- Block I: Intramural health care
- Block II: Extramural health care
- Block III: Preventive health care
- Block IV: Supply of Medical goods
- Block V: Other services, consisting of Research & Development, Education & Training and Administration.

Block I deals with the provisions and activities in the intramural health care sector. This expression "intramural" can be described as health care for patients formally admitted for a period more than 24 hours. As can be seen from the description however this expression does not differ much from the expression in-patient care used by the OECD. "In-patient" care is described as all institutions providing acute hospital care, psychiatric care, nursing home care, home care and some forms of long term care (e.g. rehabilitation, post clinical care, specialised chronic facilities in which (para)medical care constitutes a substantial part of total outlays). Another expression used in the international literature is "stationary" care.

Although the contents of all the expressions is more or less the same, none of the expressions covers the contents completely and uniquely. In the continuation of this report the subjects will indicated by the Block numbers as mentioned above. For reasons of readability the terms listed in the Block list are mentioned as well.

Ceteris paribus the same reasoning is valid for the expressions "extramural" health care, "out-patient" health care and "ambulatory" care. Although the contents of these words is more or less synonymous these expressions are replaced by Block II.

On analogy to Block I and II we chose for Block III (on Prevention) and Blocks IV (on Medical goods) and Block V (on Other services).

In creating country comparisons the need for embedding them in a larger framework is apparent. This larger framework was found in the OECD health statistics. As financial data are presented in local currency units a common basis is needed for the presentation of the data. Any comparison not limited to a quotient of two phenomena (e.g. percentages, etc.), creates the need for common denominators. PPP's (Purchasing Power Parities) can be used as denominators. In this comparison PPP's are used as denominators to recalculate Gross Domestic Product (GDP). The PPP of GDP however is not very usable for a small part of the GDP, e.g. health care. For every sector in the economy a PPP must be composed and calculated. The basket of goods and services and their prices, created for health care services is still being discussed in the European Union. Therefore PPP's are only used in relation to the GDP.

Another more commonly used deflator to create comparable data in absolute terms is the dollar exchange rate for local currency units. Due to the volatility of the dollar in recent years any intertemporal comparison has its limitations. For a comparison between countries limited to a one year period the dollar exchange rate is very usable. The advantage of the US dollar is that it is an internationally accepted measuring and calculation unit.

Within Europe a third deflator is available, the ECU. Although, being a composite measuring unit, this is less volatile than the US dollar, its limited actual use in the international economy is a disadvantage. In the bilateral comparisons the US dollar exchange rate is used as a common basis. The OECD supplies recent data on e.g. health care expenditures, GDP, PPP and exchange rates. These data have been supplemented by data on ECU-rates for all participating countries.

In the following paragraphs the general framework data for the participants referred to above are described. In the general framework an attempt is made to put the health care sector of a participant in perspective with the economic data. To create this perspective the data from the OECD Health Data Bank 1997 are used, not only for the data on health care but also for data on economic factors and population.

9.3.2 *The Netherlands–Denmark*

In table 9.1 below the data as supplied in the OECD Health Data Bank are presented for the Netherlands and for Denmark.

The data on GDP per capita show a remarkable difference in Denmark's favour, where the value of the production in 1995 is some 30 percent higher than in the Netherlands, measured in US dollars. Although the ECU is less volatile than the US dollar, the production in ECU is also some 30 percent higher. A theoretically better way to compare general economic data is the purchasing power parity. Measured in PPP's the production of Denmark is some 10 percent higher.

Table 9.1
Health care costs and GDP: the Netherlands–Denmark, 1995

	Netherlands	Denmark
	1995	1995
Expenditures on health care per capita (US $)	2,232	2,108
Expenditures on health care per capita (ECU)	1,711	1,611
Expenditures on health care in % of GDP	8.8	6.4
GDP per capita (US $)	25,476	33,190
GDP per capita (PPP)	19,719	21,537
GDP per capita (ECU)	19,531	25,357

Source: OECD Health Data Bank 1997.

OECD data on health care expenditures show that the expenditures on health care in the Netherlands is $ 124 per capita higher compared to Denmark. Measured in ECU the difference is still 100 ECU. The share of GDP spent on health care in Denmark, however, is also significantly smaller compared with that in the Netherlands.

9.3.3 *The Netherlands–Germany*

The data presented by the OECD for the Netherlands and comparable data for Germany show a difference in GDP per capita of 15.1 percent between the Netherlands and Germany, both production expressed in US dollars or in ECU. As GDP measured in PPP shows a difference of 5.2 percent, the comparison of the Netherlands and Germany the results is indeed influenced by the choice of deflator: US $ or PPP.

Table 9.2
Health care costs and GDP: the Netherlands–Germany, 1994

	Netherlands	Germany
	1994	1994
Expenditures on health care per capita (US $)	1,923	2,581
Expenditures on health care per capita (ECU)	1,621	2,178
Expenditures on health care in % of GDP	8.8	10.3
GDP per capita (US $)	21,876	25,173
GDP per capita (PPP)	18,709	19,700
GDP per capita (ECU)	18,449	21,239

Source: OECD Health Data Bank 1997.

Comparing the data presented by the for the Netherlands and Germany shows an expenditure on health per capita in the Netherlands of $ 1,923 in 1994 against $ 2,581 in Germany, a difference: of $ 658 per capita. Expressed in ECU the difference is also great; ECU 557. The share of health care expenditures in German GDP is 1.5 percentage points more than in the Netherlands (Germany 10.3 percent and the Netherlands 8.8 percent of GDP).

9.3.4 *The Netherlands–France*

GDP per capita for France is 3.9 percent higher than GDP per capita in the Netherlands, expressed in US dollars. In ECU the difference is 3.6 percent. Measured in purchasing power the GDP of France compared with the Netherlands differs by 1.2 percent. So for the bilateral comparison between the Netherlands and France it is of little or no importance whether US dollars or PPP's are used as a deflator.

According to the OECD Health Data Bank France spent 2,616 dollars per capita on health care in 1995 compared with 2,232 dollars in the Netherlands. In France 16 percent more is spent on health (per capita). Measured as a share of GDP the difference between the two countries is more remarkable. In the Netherlands 8.8 percent is spent on health compared with 9.9 percent in France, a difference of 1.1 percentage point.

Table 9.3
Health care costs and GDP: the Netherlands–France, 1995

	Netherlands	France
	1995	1995
Expenditures on health care per capita (US $)	2,232	2,616
Expenditures on health care per capita (ECU)	1,711	1,999
Expenditures on health care in % of GDP	8.8	9.9
GDP per capita (US $)	25,476	26,470
GDP per capita (PPP)	19,719	19,953
GDP per capita (ECU)	19,531	20,228

Source: OECD Health Data Bank 1997.

9.3.5 The Netherlands–Switzerland

For the comparison of health care costs and general data based on the OECD Health Data Bank in the Netherlands and Switzerland data on 1994 and 1995 the following summarised data are available.

Table 9.4
Health care costs and GDP: the Netherlands–Switzerland, 1994, 1995

	Netherlands		Switzerland	
	1994	1995	1994	1995
Expenditures on health care per capita (US $)	1,923	2,232	3,496	4,210
Expenditures on health care per capita (ECU)	1,621	1,711	2,956	3,205
Expenditures on health care in % of GDP	8.8	8.8	9.6	9.8
GDP per capita (US $)	21,896	25,476	36,607	42,811
GDP per capita (PPP)	18,709	19,719	23,882	24,523
GDP per capita (ECU)	18,449	19,531	30,958	35,592

Source: OECD Health Data Bank 1997.

The data on GDP (US $) show a remarkable difference. GDP per capita in Switzerland is almost 68 percent higher than in the Netherlands (both in 1994 and in 1995). This remarkable difference does not change by expressing the GDP in ECU. Still the gap in production between Switzerland and the Netherlands is 68 percent. A large part of this difference might be explained by Switzerland's strong position in the international money markets, a position reflected in the exchange rates of the Swiss franc and Dutch guilder respectively to the dollar. GDP calculated in PPP's still shows a difference in favour of the Swiss economy, but the difference is reduced to some 25 percent.

No PPP's are available to deflate health care expenditures specifically, so all the data on health care are presented in US $. In Switzerland almost double the amount is spent on health per capita compared to the Netherlands ($ 4,210 in Switzerland in 1995 to $ 2,232 in the Netherlands in that same year). Health care calculated as a percentage share in GDP shows a difference of 1.0 percentage points spent more in Switzerland than in the Netherlands.

9.3.6 *The Netherlands–Belgium*

For Belgium and the Netherlands data on 1994 and 1995 are presented below.

Table 9.5
Health care costs and GDP: the Netherlands–Belgium, 1994, 1995

	Netherlands		Belgium	
	1994	1995	1994	1995
Expenditures on health care per capita (US $)	1,923	2,232	1,845	2,126
Expenditures on health care per capita (ECU)	1,621	1,711	1,557	1,627
Expenditures on health care in % of GDP	8.8	8.8	8.1	8.0
GDP per capita (US $)	21,896	25,476	22,684	26,564
GDP per capita (PPP)	18,709	19,719	20,316	20,814
GDP per capita (ECU)	18,449	19,531	19,338	20,328

Source: OECD Health Data Bank 1997.

GDP per capita in Belgium is 4.3 percent higher expressed in US dollars than in the Netherlands in 1995. In ECU GDP of Belgium exceeds the GDP of the Netherlands by 4.1 percent. Measured in purchasing power the GDP of Belgium compared with the Netherlands differs 5.5 percent in 1995. So for the bilateral comparison between the Netherlands and Belgium it is of little or no importance whether US dollars or PPP's are used as a deflator.

According to the OECD Health Data Bank 2,126 dollars per capita was spent on health care in 1995 in Belgium and $ 2,232 in the Netherlands a difference of 106 dollars per capita. Measured as a share of GDP the difference between the two countries is more remarkable. In the Netherlands 8.8 percent is spent on health compared to 8.0 percent in Belgium, a difference of 0.8 percentage point.

To clarify these differences comparable sets of activities were constructed for all participating countries. In comparing these sets of activities it should be kept in mind that the contents of the various Blocks supplied for the project is different from the one supplied to the OECD.

In the following chapters the Bilateral Packages for Block I (Intramural health care), Block II (Extramural health care), Block III on Prevention, Block IV on Medical goods will be presented. In the final chapter on the construction of the Bilateral Packages (chapter 14) an attempt to create a BCP on Other services is presented.

10. Bilateral Comparable Package Block I: Intramural health care, update

10.1 Introduction

After the finishing of phase I of the project concerning Block I: Intramural health care it was decided to update the data of the provisions and activities in this Block, in order to be able to create a complete picture of the health care sector. In this chapter the updates of the data on Block I: Intramural health care are presented.

During the process of updating we noticed that if the contents of the Dutch Health Accounts would not be changed, it would be almost impossible for some countries to create Bilateral Packages. One of the reasons was that some activities that are no part of the Health Accounts in the Netherlands are implicitly included in provisions of Block I in other countries.

As a consequence of this the contents of the Health Accounts used for the Bilateral Comparisons is 'expanded'. This means that some provisions that are, largely on historical grounds, no part of the Health Accounts, are added. Abortion clinics and Institutions fore supervised dwelling are for that reason included in the data set.

Participants changed the input as well, in some cases providing a "constructed" Health Account. This constructed Health Account is used as Input in the project.

Another consequence of the updating process and the reconsidering of all activities and provisions is that the contents of Specialist's practices was changed. Some 85 percent of the total expenditures is transferred to Block I: Intramural health care and some 15 percent of the total expenditures stayed in Block II: Extramural health care.

10.2 Bilateral Comparisons 1994, 1995

10.2.1 The Netherlands–Denmark

Like in Phase I of the project the Institutions for the mentally deficient, and the Nursing homes are excluded from the Bilateral Comparisons for the Netherlands; for Denmark the Day centres for the elderly were excluded. For the Health spa's no data are supplied for 1995, although these provisions were a part of the Danish Health Accounts in 1993.

In the Netherlands during the revisions process some provisions are added to the comparable package. In the Bilateral Comparison The Netherlands - Denmark this concerns e.g. the Abortion clinics and Short term recovery homes. In phase I this provision was included in the provisions not present in the Netherlands (and is no part of the BCP).

Table 10.1
Results of the Bilateral Comparison Block I: the Netherlands–Denmark, 1995

	Netherlands	Denmark
	1995	1995
Inpatient Health care (OECD)		
Expenditures per capita (US $)	1,173	1,310
Expenditures per capita (ECU)	899	1,001
Expenditures in % of GDP	4.6	4.0
BCP expenditures on Block I: Intramural health care		
Expenditures in US $ (x 1 million)	14,986	5,810
Expenditures in ECU (x 1 million)	11,489	4,439
Expenditures per capita (US $)	968	1,112
Expenditures per capita (ECU)	742	850
Expenditures in % of GDP	3.8	3.4

In the OECD Health data bank the Netherlands reports for 1995 an amount of US $ 1,173 per capita, $ 137 per capita less than Denmark. Calculated into ECU the difference is still an amount of ECU 102. Measured as an percentage of GDP however Denmark spends 0.6 percentage points less than the Netherlands.

Contrary to what might be expected in the Bilateral Comparison the differences between the Netherlands and Denmark are larger. In US dollars the Netherlands spends $ 144 per capita less. Expressed in percentages of GDP the difference is considerably smaller, amounting to 0.6 percentage points.

Generally the results in relative terms of the update presented here are not different from the ones presented in phase I. Particularly however the Dutch side in the relative positions changed, caused by the inclusion in Block I of a large part of the specialists. The Netherlands now has a higher amount on the BCP of Block I both measured in US $ per capita and as a percentage of GDP (compared to the results in Phase I of the project).

10.2.2 The Netherlands–Germany

In the updating process in Germany some small 'errors' were eliminated in the material supplied for international comparison (e.g. in the data on the Oncological and Radiotherapeutical day treatment).

Like in the Bilateral Comparison for Denmark the Abortion clinics and the Short term recovery homes are added to the Bilateral Package concerning the Netherlands and Germany.

In this Phase of the project, like in Phase I, the Institutions for the mentally deficient (along with some smaller provisions) are excluded form the comparisons for the Netherlands. For Germany the expenditures on the Health spas are not included in the Bilateral Comparison, like all different kinds of treatment for the disabled and handicapped.

Table 10.2
Results of the Bilateral Comparison Block I: the Netherlands–Germany, 1994

	Netherlands	Germany
	1994	1994
Inpatient Health care (OECD)		
Expenditures per capita (US $)	1,007	939
Expenditures per capita (ECU)	848	793
Expenditures in % of GDP	4.6	3.7
BCP expenditures on Block I: Intramural health care		
Expenditures in US $ (x 1 million)	15,688	92,286
Expenditures in ECU (x 1 million)	13,219	77,866
Expenditures per capita (US $)	1,020	1,133
Expenditures per capita (ECU)	859	956
Expenditures in % of GDP	4.7	4.5

Comparing OECD Health data bank data the differences in expenditures on inpatient care are rather small. Germany spends $ 68 per capita less compared to the Netherlands. If the expenditures are expressed as a share of GDP the difference between the Netherlands and Germany is almost one percentage point.

In the Bilateral Package on Block I the difference between the Netherlands and Germany is $ 113 per capita, but contrary to the data in the OECD data now the

Netherlands spend less than Germany. The gap between the Netherlands and Germany, expressed in a percentage of GDP is diminished and amounts to 0.2 percentagepoint.

The differences between Germany and the Netherlands are less pronounced due to the fact that a share of the Specialists expenditures is moved from Block II: Extramural health to Block I: Intramural health for the Netherlands.

10.2.3 The Netherlands–France

The third comparison is made for the Netherlands and France. France updated the data for 1993. At the same time France supplied the data for 1994 and 1995.

However for the BCP it is not possible to present both 1994 and 1995 for France (and for the Netherlands), due to the fact that data on provisions to be transferred from other Blocks to Block I for 1994 are lacking. This means that the construction of the BCP the Netherlands–France is limited to 1995.

For the Netherlands the Institutions for the mentally deficient are not included in the comparison, as are some other small provisions. Because however in France the nursing home activity is to a large extent not included, the Nursing homes are excluded form the bilateral comparison for the Netherlands. For France, the health spas are not included.

Table 10.3
Results of the Bilateral Comparison Block I: the Netherlands–France, 1995

	Netherlands	France
	1995	1995
Inpatient Health care (OECD)		
Expenditures per capita (US $)	1,173	1,163
Expenditures per capita (ECU)	899	889
Expenditures in % of GDP	4.6	4.4
BCP expenditures on Block I: Intramural health care		
Expenditures in US $ (x 1 million)	14,355	67,732
Expenditures in ECU (x 1 million)	11,006	51,758
Expenditures per capita (US $)	927	1,166
Expenditures per capita (ECU)	711	891
Expenditures in % of GDP	3.6	4.4

The Netherlands spends US $ 1,173 per capita in 1995, just a little bit more than France (US $ 1,163) according to the data supplied tot the OECD. Contrary to the expectations in the composition of the Bilateral Package the differences are greater.

In France $ 239 per capita is spend more on Block I than in the Netherlands in 1995. Measured in percentages of GDP in France in 1995 just 1.2 percentage point was spent more on intramural health care in comparison to the Netherlands.

10.2.4 The Netherlands–Switzerland

Switzerland supplied for the update on the data two years as well, 1994 and 1995.

In the process of creating comparability on Block I for the Netherlands only a very small part of Block I activities had to be deducted. This deduction concerns an amount of $ 37 million for both 1994 and 1995. Due to the fact that the Statistical Office of Switzerland supplied separate data on the nursing home activity, there is no need to include the Homes for the elderly in the Bilateral Comparison for the Netherlands. On the other hand no calculation for the Homes for the elderly for Switzerland was necessary; the amount supplied for this activity is not included in the comparison for Switzerland.

Table 10.4
Results of the Bilateral Comparison Block I: the Netherlands–Switzerland, 1994, 1995

	Netherlands		Switzerland	
	1994	1995	1994	1995
Inpatient Health care (OECD)				
Expenditures per capita (US $)	1,007	1,173	1,794	2,176
Expenditures per capita (ECU)	848	899	1,518	1,657
Expenditures in % of GDP	4.6	4.6	4.9	5.1
BCP expenditures on Block I: Intramural health care				
Expenditures in US $ (x 1 million)	17,030	20,073	13,147	15,720
Expenditures in ECU (x 1 million)	14,349	15,389	11,119	11,968
Expenditures per capita (US $)	1,107	1,297	1,868	2,194
Expenditures per capita (ECU)	933	994	1,580	1,670
Expenditures in % of GDP	5.1	5.1	5.1	5.1

The differences – according to the OECD – in amounts spend on Block I provisions is absolutely the largest between the Netherlands and Switzerland. In 1994 the difference is $ 787 per capita and in 1995 US $ 1,003 is spend more in Switzerland than in the Netherlands.

In absolute amounts the BCP Netherlands–Switzerland is the largest. This is caused by the fact that in this comparison the Institutions for the mentally deficient are included. In US $ this provision is accountable for 3,300 million US $ in 1995, or 9 percent of the total bilateral package of the Netherlands.

The differences in spending per capita on Block I are smaller compared to the OECD data, but are still quite large; $ 761 in 1994 and $ 897 in 1995. Expressed in percentages of GDP the Swiss spend just as much as the Dutch on Block I provisions (5.1 percent).

Comparing 1994 and 1995 it is remarkable that measured in percentages of GDP both in the Netherlands and Switzerland the share stayed the same.
Expressed in ECU the Dutch spent in 1995 ECU 61 more than in 1994, while the Swiss spend some ECU 90 per capita more.

10.2.5 The Netherlands–Belgium

Belgium like Switzerland and France supplied data on Block I provisions for two years, 1994 and 1995.

Only for the Netherlands some provisions are excluded from the comparison. The most important being the Institutions for the mentally deficient.

Table 10.5
Results of the Bilateral Comparison Block I: the Netherlands–Belgium, 1994, 1995

	Netherlands		Belgium	
	1994	1995	1994	1995
Inpatient Health care (OECD)				
Expenditures per capita (US $)	1,007	1,173	664	794
Expenditures per capita (ECU)	848	899	560	608
Expenditures in % of GDP	4.6	4.6	2.9	3.0
BCP expenditures on Block I: Intramural health care				
Expenditures in US $ (x 1 million)	15,158	17,855	8,213	9,859
Expenditures in ECU (x 1 million)	12,772	13,689	6,929	7,545
Expenditures per capita (US $)	985	1,153	812	974
Expenditures per capita (ECU)	830	884	685	745
Expenditures in % of GDP	4.5	4.5	3.6	3.7

For the project Belgium supplied a large data set that made it possible to calculate Hospital expenditures which are better comparable with the other countries. In Belgium a lot of expenditures generated in hospitals are listed under the physicians

headings. The same is true for the expenditures of the physician share in the expenditures of out-patient departments.
The last item that has to be mentioned here is the item on Additional expenditures containing the out-of-pocket expenditures and the voluntary supplementary insurance. These additional information of course influences the (in)comparability of the OECD data on Inpatient care and the data as presented in the Bilateral Comparison.

In Belgium the smallest absolute amount (of the six participating countries) is spend on inpatient health care according to the data supplied by the OECD. This is true for the amounts per capita and for the percentages of GDP in 1994 and in 1995.

In the Bilateral Packages of Block I these large differences are gone to a large extent. In the BCP of Block I the Belgians spends $ 173 per capita less in 1994 and $ 179 (in 1995) less on these provisions compared to the Netherlands. Also expressed in percentages of GDP it is clear that the contents of Block I is different from the contents on inpatient care supplied to the OECD.

10.3 *Summary of the Bilateral Comparisons on Block I: Intramural health care*

In this paragraph the summary of the previous Bilateral Packages is presented for the Netherlands, Germany, France, Switzerland, Denmark and Belgium. Four countries supplied data for 1994 (the Netherlands, Germany, Switzerland and Belgium), five countries supplied data for 1995 (the Netherlands, Switzerland, Denmark, France and Belgium).

Belgium and Denmark (see table 10.6, page 148) show a smaller share of their GDP spent on Block I provisions compared to the Netherlands. In France the share of GDP devoted to Block I is larger than the share of GDP spent by the Netherlands. In Germany and Switzerland the difference with the is negligible small (in rounded numbers even zero).

Finally the data in the bilateral comparisons are presented expressed in US $ per capita and in ECU per capita (see table 10.7, page 148).

From every Bilateral Comparison it turns out that the Netherlands spends less per capita on intramural health than the other countries. The exception being Belgium. For Belgium $ 173 per capita is spent less compared to the Netherlands in 1994. In 1995 this difference is $ 179 per capita. The difference is relatively small in the bilateral package with Germany and Denmark (about US $ 100 per capita). In comparison with France the difference is $ 139 and with Switzerland (1995) the difference is approximately $ 900 per capita.

Table 10.6
Bilateral Comparison Summary on Block I: Intramural health care (% of GDP)

	OECD Inpatient care		Bilateral Comparable Package Block I		
		Difference [1]	Netherlands	Other country	Difference [1]
Year 1994					
The Netherlands	4.6				
Germany (BCP Netherlands–Germany)	3.7	–0.9	4.6	4.5	–0.1
Switzerland (BCP Netherlands–Switzerland)	4.9	0.3	5.1	5.1	0.0
Belgium (BCP Netherlands–Belgium)	2.9	–1.7	3.6	2.0	–0.9
Year 1995					
The Netherlands	4.6				
Denmark (BCP Netherlands–Denmark)	4.0	–0.6	3.8	3.4	–0.4
France (BCP Netherlands–France)	4.4	–0.2	3.6	4.4	0.8
Switzerland (BCP Netherlands–Switzerland)	5.1	0.5	5.1	5.1	0.0
Belgium (BCP Netherlands–Belgium)	3.0	–1.6	4.5	3.7	–0.8

[1] Difference in percentagepoints with respect to the Netherlands.

Table 10.7
Bilateral Comparison Summary on Block I: Intramural health care (US $ & ECU per capita)

	Year	Expenditures per capita Block I	
		US $	Ecu
The Netherlands	1995	968	742
Denmark		1,112	850
The Netherlands	1994	1,020	859
Germany		1,133	956
The Netherlands	1995	927	711
France		1,166	891
The Netherlands	1994	1,107	933
Switzerland		1,868	1,580
The Netherlands	1995	1,297	994
Switzerland		2,194	1,670
The Netherlands	1994	985	830
Belgium		812	685
The Netherlands	1995	1,153	884
Belgium		974	745

11. The Bilateral Comparable Package Block II: Extramural health care

11.1 Introduction

In this chapter Block II: Extramural health care provisions is discussed. Based on the data supplied, it is very difficult to separate Block II: Extramural and Block III: Preventive health care; the health care provisions in Blocks II and Block III are intertwined, even if only the preventive activities of provisions that are separately listed in the Health Accounts are taken into account. One of the problems is that some countries include these activities in Block II while others include them in Block III.

It may be clear that the comparability of Block II as presented in this paragraph and the comparability of Block III provisions as such is smaller than the comparability of Block II: Extramural and Block III: Preventive health care provisions together.

Still an attempt is made to separate extramural and preventive health care. The starting point is the division in provisions as presented in the questionnaires used for the project. Only in a limited number of cases an attempt is made to reclassify provisions (taking out provisions from Block II and including them in Block III for example). Unless otherwise stated it is assumed that the main activities listed as Block II are in extramural health care, and preventive activities are additional to their main activity.

Contrary to the description of Block I (in chapter 10), the description starts with some peculiarities of Dutch health care followed by the bilateral packages for the participating countries: Netherlands, Denmark, Germany, France, Switzerland and Belgium.

11.2 The Netherlands

Peculiarities of the Dutch extramural health care system concern the Specialists' practices, Health centres, Podotherapists and the Institutions for domiciliary health and social services.

Specialists' practices

Many Dutch specialists are as self-employed, for their own account, even if they are working solely in a hospital or other Block I: intramural health facilities. All the expenditures of these practices are accounted for in the extramural health care in the Dutch Health Accounts.

Noting however the description of Block II and Block I , the specialists working in the institutions should be included in the calculated accounts of the institutions. The expenditures of specialists' practices are adapted in the Dutch tables for this phenomenon. About 14% of the total expenditures of self-employed specialists is attributed to Block II; the rest (86 %) is included in Block I.

Health centres
The expenditures accounted for in this category are just the additional expenditures on top of the expenditures of the self-employed professionals (e.g. general practitioners and physiotherapists).

Podotherapists
Podotherapy is not included in the Dutch Health Accounts. For the sake of the comparability with other countries an amount is calculated based on the number of podotherapists, the average number of clients they help and the payment per session.

The institutions for domiciliary health and social services
These institutions are the result of the merger of institutions providing health care at home, maternity care, and home help. The total expenditures of these institutions were divided in a part on home/district nursing, maternity home care and home help.

11.3 Bilateral Comparisons

11.3.1 The Netherlands–Denmark

In Denmark out of pocket expenditures in the field of health care are not all included in the Health Accounts but included in the private consumption expenditures. For the project, Denmark supplied an amount for out of pocket expenditures for three categories of health professionals, i.e. General practitioners, Specialists and Dentists. There is no information on the existence of out of pocket expenditures in other categories of care.

A calculated amount for the Dental appliances is added to the Dentists practices, because in Denmark these expenditures are included in the Therapeutic appliances.

The expenditures for Speech therapists are included in the Municipal health and social services in Denmark. Although the expenditures of Municipal health and social services are not supplied separately as such, the amount of expenditures for this category of provider is included.

Health centres are not present in the Health Accounts in Denmark as is the case for Dental hygienists and Family care of mental patients. It is assumed that the activities are included in Municipal health and General practitioners, respectively Dentists and Psychiatric care. Anthroposofic health care is non existent in Denmark, in the Netherlands however these activities are not included in the Health Accounts, so for the Bilateral Comparison and the BCP this category is no problem.

In the table below, the data resulting from the Bilateral Comparison the Netherlands–Denmark are presented as well as the data from the OECD Health Data Bank 1997. The data on ambulatory care however are not limited to data on Block II but included are Block III provisions as well

Table 11.1
Results of the Bilateral Comparison Block II: the Netherlands–Denmark, 1995

	Netherlands	Denmark
	1995	1995
Ambulatory Health care (OECD) [1]		
Expenditures per capita (US $)	628	398
Expenditures per capita (ECU)	481	304
Expenditures in % of GDP	2.47	1.20
BCP expenditures on Block II: Extramural health care		
Expenditures in US $ (x 1 million)	7,302	2,805
Expenditures in ECU (x 1 million)	5,598	2,143
Expenditures per capita (US $)	472	537
Expenditures per capita (ECU)	362	410
Expenditures in % of GDP	1.85	1.62

1) Contents of Ambulatory care is different from the contents of Block II.

The OECD description of ambulatory health care includes the expenditures of the institutions in the field of prevention. The BCP includes only those providers listed in the questionnaire as being working in Block II: Extramural health care.

The difference between the OECD data on ambulatory care between the Netherlands and Denmark ($ 230 per capita) is much greater than the difference in BCP on Block II health care between the two countries (only $ 65 per capita). This is caused by differences in the contents of the package under consideration between the health accounts of the Netherlands presented to the OECD and that of Denmark. The contents of the packages supplied in the project however are quite similar.

11.3.2 The Netherlands–Germany

Germany supplied a very detailed set of data. The activities of Health centres are included in Specialists' practices although the provision is not present in Germany.

Dieticians are combined with Speech therapists; Podotherapists with Physiotherapists and Dental hygienists are included in Dentists practices. Alternative medical treatment is supplied by General practitioners and ambulatory mental health care is supplied by Psychotherapists.
Dental laboratories are included in the expenditures of Therapeutic appliances (under dentures). For comparability reasons these expenditures are transferred to Block II under the heading of Dental practices.

Table 11.2
Results of the Bilateral Comparison Block II: the Netherlands–Germany, 1994

	Netherlands	Germany
	1994	1994
Ambulatory Health care (OECD) [1]		
Expenditures per capita (US $)	550	771
Expenditures per capita (ECU)	464	650
Expenditures in % of GDP	2.51	3.06
BCP expenditures on Block II: Extramural health care		
Expenditures in US $ (x 1 million)	6,452	67,350
Expenditures in ECU (x 1 million)	5,437	56,827
Expenditures per capita (US $)	419	827
Expenditures per capita (ECU)	353	698
Expenditures in % of GDP	1.92	3.29

[1] Contents of Ambulatory care is different from the contents of Block II.

As already noted in the bilateral comparisons on Block I: intramural health care (in chapter 10, and the publication on phase I) the importance of Block II or ambulatory health care is much greater in Germany than in the Netherlands. The difference between the two countries in OECD data is $ 221 per capita or 0.5 percentage points in GDP.

The difference is even bigger in the Bilateral Comparison. In US dollars per capita Germany spends $ 408 per person more than the Netherlands; which is almost double the amount spent in the Netherlands on Block II. Expressed in ECU the difference between Germany and the Netherlands is ECU 345 per capita.

The relative importance of Block II health care in Germany can also be seen in the amount spent expressed in a percentage of GDP. In Germany 3.3 percent is spend on Block II health, compared with 1.9 percent in the Netherlands.

11.3.3 *The Netherlands–France*

In France no distinction is made between the General practitioners and Specialists since they are one class of health care providers no separate data are available. The Dispensaries (dispensaires) are taken together with the health centres. Dental hygienist are included in the Dental practices. Like Denmark France has no Anthroposofic medical treatment; professionals providing alternative medicines although known, are not included in the Health Accounts.

In France the institutions providing Family care to mental patients and Home help are not accounted for in the Health Accounts but are part of the social services; no data on these provisions are supplied. In the Bilateral Comparison these provisions are left out.

Maternity home care in France is supplied by the Mother and child protection centres. The data on this provision are supplied in the preventive health care list of provisions. The last difficulty in the comparison between the Netherlands and France is posed by the other ambulatory mental health care. Although known in France and included in the Ambulatory health care (les soins ambulatoires) it is hard to distinguish the data on this category of institution because no data are supplied for this type of provision. Based on assumptions and supplementary data by France calculations for this activity could be made

The data supplied give the following summary table on the Bilateral Comparison of the Netherlands and France for 1995.

Table 11.3
Results of the Bilateral Comparison Block II: the Netherlands–France, 1995

	Netherlands	France
	1995	1995
Ambulatory Health care (OECD) [1] [2]		
Expenditures per capita (US $)	628	604
Expenditures per capita (ECU)	481	510
Expenditures in % of GDP	2.51	2.63
BCP expenditures on Block II: Extramural health care		
Expenditures in US $ (x 1 million)	5,925	41,294
Expenditures in ECU (x 1 million)	4,542	31,555
Expenditures per capita (US $)	383	711
Expenditures per capita (ECU)	293	543
Expenditures in % of GDP	1.50	2.68

1) Contents of Ambulatory care is different from the contents of Block II.
2) OECD Data for France relate to 1994.

Unfortunately the OECD supplied no data on ambulatory health care for France for 1995 so for the comparison between the Netherlands and France concerning OECD data, 1994 data for France is used as a proxy. Using OECD data, in France 0.1 percentage point more is spent on Block II health care than in the Netherlands. Measured in US $ per capita the French spent $ 604 in 1994; just $ 24 less than the Netherlands per capita according to data supplied to the OECD.

In the Bilateral Package (on Block II) the difference in percentage of GDP spent on health between the Netherlands and France is 1.2 percentage point. In US $ France spent $ 328 per capita more on Block II health care than the Netherlands.

11.3.4 The Netherlands–Switzerland

In Switzerland, like in France, no separation was made between General practitioners and Specialists. Dental hygienists are included in the Dental practices, at least financial. Maternity home care is not included in the Health Accounts of Switzerland.

A peculiarity of the Swiss health system is the existence of the category Other ambulatory health care (without SPITEX [1)]); a provider that supplies a enormous amount of different activities. This category includes the following provisions, included in Block II in other countries: Speech therapists, Dieticians, Podotherapist, Psychotherapist, Family care of mental patients, Alternative medical treatment and Transport of patients Finally the Other ambulatory mental health care is partly integrated in the Other ambulatory health care.

To make the problem of comparing of Switzerland with all the other participants even greater, some or even all expenditures on Therapeutic appliances are included in the expenditures on Other ambulatory health care; expenditures which are included in Block IV: Medical goods in other countries.

Since a single Swiss provider combines so many activities, we tried to list and compare the same set of activities in the other participating countries.
It is obvious that for a lot of providers/activities assumptions had to made to get the data for this comparison.

In Switzerland the expenditure of the provisions Other ambulatory care amounts to $ 57 per capita. In France an equivalent number of provisions amount to $ 160 per capita.

This leaves the fact that the amount in US·$ per capita for Switzerland is very low compared to the other countries, especially if taken into account that many or maybe all Therapeutic appliances are included as well.

For the Bilateral Comparison the amount supplied for Other ambulatory services is included into the Bilateral Comparison on Block II. A calculation for the expenditures on Therapeutic appliances is made. This amount is transferred from Block II to Block III, to reduce the inequalities with the other participants.
A final remark on Switzerland concerns the fact that Switzerland supplied data for two years; both 1994 and 1995. A Bilateral Comparison is made for these two years.

Table 11.4
Results of the Bilateral Comparison Block II: the Netherlands–Switzerland, 1994, 1995

	Netherlands		Switzerland	
	1994	1995	1994	1995
Ambulatory Health care (OECD) 1)				
Expenditures per capita (US $)	550	628	1,317	1,537
Expenditures per capita (ECU)	464	481	1,114	1,197
Expenditures in % of GDP	2.51	2.47	3.60	3.67
BCP expenditures on Block II: Extramural health care				
Expenditures in US $ (x 1 million)	6,193	7,087	7,009	8,577
Expenditures in ECU (x 1 million)	5,218	5,434	5,927	6,529
Expenditures per capita (US $)	403	458	996	1,197
Expenditures per capita (ECU)	339	351	842	911
Expenditures in % of GDP	1.84	1.80	2.72	2.80

1) Contents of Ambulatory care is different from the contents of Block II.

There is an enormous difference between Switzerland and the Netherlands as is shown by the data presented by the OECD and the data supplied for the project.

In the Bilateral Comparable package expressed in US $ per capita the Netherlands spend $ 403 and Switzerland $ 996 per capita in 1994, that is $ 593 difference. In the OECD data the difference between the Netherlands and Switzerland is much larger for 1994 ($ 558 versus $ 1,140).

Looking at the detailed data supplied by Switzerland, the explanation for the difference in the BCP can be found to a large extent in the medical professions (General practitioner and Specialist) on which over $ 2,000 million more is spent in Switzerland than in the Netherlands.

Due to the fact that Switzerland supplied data for two years on this subject it is possible to make some remarks on the comparison of these two years. In the Bilateral Comparable Package of 1995 Switzerland spends some 10 percent more expressed in ECU than in 1994. The Netherlands on the other hand spend some 4 percent more.

The expenditures per capita show the same picture; the expenditures in Switzerland grew by 8 percent, in the Netherlands by 4 percent.

11.3.5 The Netherlands–Belgium

The last comparison concerns the Netherlands and Belgium. Belgium supplied an extensive data set trying to distinguish as many activities as possible.

Due to the fact that no division of the out of pocket expenditures for the various Blocks are available in Belgium some calculations were necessary. The same holds true for the expenditures of the voluntary health insurance and some small subsidies (e.g. from the central government). The total of these expenditures are listed under the heading of Additional payments.

For the activities on Transport of patients, calculations were necessary e.g. on the expenditures of ordered transport. The same is true for the home help expenditures: the social part of Home care is calculated and added to the data on Home help in the health care field. Out-patient departments were separated from Physicians expenditures and transferred to Block I comparisons, and finally the expenditures on Dental prostheses were transferred from Block IV: Medical goods to Dentist practices (in Block II).

Below the results of the Bilateral Comparison are presented. These data are supplemented by data from the OECD as was the case for all the other countries. Because Belgium supplied data for two years (1994 and 1995) the table below contains data on these two years.

Table 11.5
Results of the Bilateral Comparison Block II: the Netherlands–Belgium, 1994, 1995

	Netherlands		Belgium	
	1994	1995	1994	1995
Ambulatory Health care (OECD) [1]				
Expenditures per capita (US $)	550	628	674	801
Expenditures per capita (ECU)	464	481	569	613
Expenditures in % of GDP	2.51	2.47	2.97	3.02
BCP expenditures on Block II: Extramural health care				
Expenditures in US $ (x 1 million)	6,444	7,371	4,556	5,470
Expenditures in ECU (x 1 million)	5,430	5,651	3,844	4,186
Expenditures per capita (US $)	419	476	450	540
Expenditures per capita (ECU)	353	365	380	413
Expenditures in % of GDP	1.91	1.87	1.99	2.03

[1] Contents of Ambulatory care is different from the contents of Block II.

In the OECD health data bank Belgium supplied an amount of $ 674 per capita in 1994, the Netherlands $ 550 per capita on Block II. The difference between the Netherlands and Belgium results in $ 124 spend more in Belgium per capita in 1994.

In the Bilateral comparisons the difference between Belgium and the Netherlands is $ 31 per capita in 1994 and $ 64 in 1995.

For Belgium as well as for Switzerland two years of data are available. Belgium spent some 9 percent more in 1995 than in 1994 on the BCP expressed in ECU The Netherlands some 4 percent. In Belgium the expenditures in ECU per capita expanded by 9 percent as well; for the Netherlands however the growth per capita was limited to 3 percent.

11.4 *Summary on the Bilateral Comparisons on Block II health care*

In this paragraph a summary of the results of the five Bilateral Comparisons is presented for the six countries: the Netherlands, Denmark, Germany, France and Switzerland. Three countries supplied data for 1994 (Germany, Switzerland and Belgium) and four for 1995 (Denmark, France, Switzerland and Belgium).

Table 11.6
Bilateral Comparison Summary on Block II: Extramural health care (% of GDP)

	OECD[2) 3)] Ambulatory care		Bilateral Comparable Package Block II		
		Difference[1)]	Nether-lands	Other country	Difference[1)]
Year 1994					
The Netherlands	2.51				
Germany (BCP Netherlands–Germany)	3.06	0.49	1.92	3.29	1.37
Switzerland (BCP Netherlands–Switzerland)	3.60	1.09	1.84	2.72	0.88
Belgium (BCP Netherlands–Belgium)	2.97	0.46	1.91	1.99	0.08
Year 1995					
The Netherlands	2.47				
Denmark (BCP Netherlands–Denmark)	1.20	-1.27	1.85	1.62	-0.23
France (BCP Netherlands–France)	2.63	0.16	1.50	2.68	1.18
Switzerland (BCP Netherlands–Switzerland)	3.67	1.20	1.80	2.80	1.00
Belgium (BCP Netherlands–Belgium)	3.02	0.82	1.87	2.03	0.16

1) Difference in percentagepoints with respect to the Netherlands.
2) Contents of Ambulatory care is different from the contents of Block II.
3) OECD Data for France relate to 1994.

Only Denmark has a smaller share of GDP devoted to Block II health care than the Netherlands in the OECD data bank; for all other countries the share of Block II in GDP is larger.
The same is true with respect to the BCP, although the difference between the Netherlands and Denmark diminished to 0.23 percent. This is roughly one sixth of the difference compared to the data in the OECD data bank.

For three participants the difference with respect to the Netherlands in the BCP on Block II is around 1 percentage point; i.e. Germany, Switzerland and France. In the comparison with Belgium the differences are very small.
A part of the explanation is found in the way the expenditures of Specialists' practices are treated in the Dutch data. Because almost all specialists are as self-employed professionals working in hospitals, about 85 percent of the total expenditures is added to Block I in the comparison and is no longer a part of Block II expenditures. Below the summary of the data is provided calculated in US·$ per capita and in ECU per capita.

Table 11.7
Bilateral Comparison Summary on Block II: Extramural health care (US $ & ECU per capita

	Year	Expenditures per capita Block II	
		US $	Ecu
The Netherlands	1995	472	362
Denmark		537	410
The Netherlands	1994	419	353
Germany		827	698
The Netherlands	1995	383	293
France		711	543
The Netherlands	1994	403	339
Switzerland		996	842
The Netherlands	1995	458	351
Switzerland		1,197	911
The Netherlands	1994	419	353
Belgium		450	380
The Netherlands	1995	476	365
Belgium		540	413

Some additional remarks can be made. Measured in US $ per capita the amount spent by the Netherlands is $ 31 lower than in Belgium (1994) and $ 65 lower than in Denmark; all other Bilateral Comparisons show a remarkably different picture. In all other countries the amount spent per capita is at least $ 300 more in comparison to the Netherlands; in Switzerland some $ 600 more in 1994, caused by a much larger amount spent on Physicians (General practitioner and Specialist) in Switzerland.

The explanation for the low Danish data might be the fact that out of pocket expenditures are not regularly included in the health accounts and that due to this fact some out of pocket expenditures are not included in the bilateral comparison the Netherlands - Denmark. Another part of the explanation might be that provisions categorised as Block II health care are listed as preventive health care (Block III) or Block I: Intramural health care in Denmark. Further research is necessary to explain this difference in data.

Note

1) SPITEX means hospital care supplied outside the hospital; a form of home care.

12. Bilateral Comparable Package Block III: Prevention

12.1 Introduction

It turned out to be very difficult to separate Block II: Extramural health care provisions and preventive health care provisions. Although it might be possible to create a complete separation in activities, in financial terms it is complicated if not impossible. So as far as the data allow it, a separation of preventive care provisions is made and presented in this chapter.

Below, the five Bilateral Comparisons are presented. First, however, a description of the peculiarities of the Dutch health care with respect to preventive activities (provisions).

12.2 The Netherlands

Some remarks are in order on the activities concerning health education and information, the fight against alcoholism and drugs, prevention of accidents, mass screening on risk factors and genetic counselling.

Health education and information is not performed in an independent provision. This activity is included in activities of all health care providers – as it is in all other countries. It can be also seen as one of the main activities of Institutions providing domiciliary health and social services and in the Municipal health services.

Although the Treatment of alcoholism and drugs is a separate activity in the Netherlands no official data are available on the prevention category of the Fight against alcohol and drug abuse. It is assumed however, that the largest part of the expenditures in this field are accounted for by these institutions. A calculation was made of the amount of expenditures responsible for the activity of prevention in this area. This amount is transferred from Block II to Block III health care on prevention.

Prevention of accidents at home and in the field of traffic activities are not counted in the Health Accounts; Prevention of accidents at work are an integral part of the Occupational health care providers. No separate data exists on the amounts spent on Mass screening on risk factors.

Genetic counselling is performed by and large in Hospitals, like in Germany and Denmark. For the Netherlands a calculation is made for the amount attributable to

Genetic counselling. This amount is deducted from Block I (the hospital sector) and transferred to Block III on prevention.

Finally activities in the field of School health and School dental health (separate provisions until the beginning of the nineties) are performed by the Municipal health services.

12.3 *Bilateral Comparisons*

The OECD presents no separate data on the field of preventive health care. These provisions are by and large included in the institutions providing ambulatory health care. A comparison of the Bilateral Package on preventive health and the OECD data on this subject is therefore not possible. In the final part of this paragraph the results of the comparisons on Block II: Extramural and Block III: Preventive health care will be added to make a comparison with the OECD data on ambulatory care possible.

Here the Bilateral Comparisons and the Bilateral Comparable Packages for preventive health care will be presented.

12.3.1 The Netherlands–Denmark

No separate data on Environmental hygiene was presented by Denmark, the data are combined with the data on Drinking water surveillance. Only one amount of expenditures was supplied for both activities.

For the Fight against smoking the data presented contain only the amounts spent by the central government, although counties and private organisations spent money on the prevention in this field as well. A calculation for these organisations is made and included in the data.

Excluded from the Bilateral Comparison is the Mass screening on risk factors on which no data are available.

Table 12.1
Results of the Bilateral Comparison Block III: the Netherlands–Denmark, 1995

	Netherlands	Denmark
	1995	1995
BCP expenditures on Block III: Preventive health care		
Expenditures in US $ (x 1 million)	1,137	522
Expenditures in ECU (x 1 million)	872	399
Expenditures per capita (US $)	73	100
Expenditures per capita (ECU)	56	76
Expenditures in % of GDP	0.29	0.30

Because many institutions active in prevention in one country are not known in the other, the amount spent on the total of the activity prevention are not big ($ 100 per capita was spent in Denmark and $ 79 in the Netherlands).

12.3.2 The Netherlands–Germany

For the Bilateral Comparison The Netherlands–Germany the activities on Environmental hygiene are excluded. No data are available on the Fight against alcohol and drug abuse; it is assumed that these data are included in other activities supplied by other providers (paid for by government and health insurance funds).

The Bilateral Comparison results on preventive health care for Germany and the Netherlands are presented below.

Table 12.2
Results of the Bilateral Comparison Block III: the Netherlands–Germany, 1994

	Netherlands	Germany
	1994	1994
BCP expenditures on Block III: Preventive health care		
Expenditures in US $ (x 1 million)	899	7,410
Expenditures in ECU (x 1 million)	757	6,253
Expenditures per capita (US $)	58	91
Expenditures per capita (ECU)	49	77
Expenditures in % of GDP	0.27	0.36

Measured in US-$ per capita Germany spent almost fifty percent on preventive activities compared to the Netherlands (at least taken prevention as a separate activity). Although measured as a percentage of GDP the difference between Germany and the Netherlands seems small, the 0.09 percentage point represents a substantial amount of money.

12.3.3 The Netherlands–France

No separate data are available on the fields of Health protection and Health promotion in France. One amount of money is supplied for both clusters of activities. It is assumed is that all activities listed separately in these two fields in the questionnaire are included in this amount [1).

Table 12.3
Results of the Bilateral Comparison Block III: the Netherlands–France, 1995

	Netherlands	France
	1995	1995
BCP expenditures on Block III: Preventive health care		
Expenditures in US $ (x 1 million)	1,137	3,238
Expenditures in ECU (x 1 million)	872	2,474
Expenditures per capita (US $)	73	56
Expenditures per capita (ECU)	56	43
Expenditures in % of GDP	0.29	0.21

In the BCP France–the Netherlands the amounts spent on preventive health care by the Netherlands is 40 percent higher compared to France, both measured in US $ per capita and as a percentage of GDP. This is all the more remarkable because the limited amount of data available on preventive health care and the assumptions made on provisions.

12.3.4 The Netherlands– Switzerland

Both Drinking water surveillance and Environmental hygiene are activities in the field of preventive health care on which no data are available for Switzerland because these provisions are not adopted in the Health Accounts. According to the Swiss data set the same holds true for the Early detection of developmental disorders.
The results of the Bilateral Comparison for the Netherlands–Switzerland for the years 1994 and 1995 is presented below.

Table 12.4
Results of the Bilateral Comparison Block III: the Netherlands–Switzerland, 1994, 1995

	Netherlands		Switzerland	
	1994	1995	1994	1995
BCP expenditures on Block III: Preventive health care				
Expenditures in US $ (x 1 million)	850	1,044	420	539
Expenditures in ECU (x 1 million)	716	800	355	410
Expenditures per capita (US $)	55	67	60	75
Expenditures per capita (ECU)	47	52	50	57
Expenditures in % of GDP	0.25	0.26	0.16	0.18

The share on preventive health care expressed as a percentage of GDP for Switzerland is low. One of the reasons for this is that many activities are performed by General practitioners and Specialists in Switzerland on which separate data are available in the Netherlands. Health education, Fight against smoking, Genetic counselling, Antenatal assessment, Mass screening on specific diseases, and Mass screening on risk factors are activities performed by General practitioners and Specialists. No calculation on the expenditures of these activities is made, because the General practitioner and the Specialist are already included in the data and the Bilateral Package on Block II: Extramural health care, and there was no information on which to base plausible assumptions for the calculation of these activities. Included in the BCP are Health education, Fight against smoking and Mass screening on specific diseases.

The more obvious is the similarity in data measured in US $ per capita. Both Switzerland and the Netherlands spend about the same amount per capita on prevention. The difference between the two countries is small ($ 5 per capita in 1994 and $ 8 in 1995).

Expressed as a percentage of GDP however the difference between the Netherlands and Switzerland was 0.09 percentage points in 1994 and 0.08 percentage points in 1995).

Comparison of the data for Switzerland and the Netherlands for 1994 and 1995 shows that expenditures (in ECU) grew by 12 percent in the Netherlands and 15 percent in Switzerland. Expressed in ECU per capita there is no difference in the growth in both countries (11 percent for the Netherlands and 14 percent for Switzerland respectively).

12.3.5 The Netherlands–Belgium

The last Bilateral Comparison prevention is made for the Netherlands and Belgium. Belgium like Switzerland supplied data for two years, 1994 and 1995.

Almost all activities were supplied by Belgium as requested. Below the results of the comparison are presented for these two years.

Table 12.5
Results of the Bilateral Comparison Block III: the Netherlands–Belgium, 1994, 1995

	Netherlands		Belgium	
	1994	1995	1994	1995
BCP expenditures on Block III: Preventive health care				
Expenditures in US $ (x 1 million)	893	1,131	333	378
Expenditures in ECU (x 1 million)	753	867	281	289
Expenditures per capita (US $)	58	73	33	37
Expenditures per capita (ECU)	49	56	28	29
Expenditures in % of GDP	0.27	0.29	0.15	0.14

Although Belgium supplied almost all activities in the field of prevention, the amount spent on the subject of prevention is rather small in comparison to the Netherlands. A possible reason is that a lot of activities are implicitly included in other providers of care in Belgium for which separate data are available (or calculated) in the Netherlands.

Because Belgium supplied data for two years (as well as Switzerland) the data for these two years can be compared. In the Netherlands the package on prevention (measured in ECU) grew by 15 percent, the same package in Belgium only by 3 percent. Measured in ECU per capita the results do not change much In the Netherlands the growth per capita was 14 percent and in Belgium only 3 percent.

12.4 *Summary of the Bilateral Comparison for Block III: Preventive health care*

In this last paragraph we present a summary on the results on Bilateral Comparisons of preventive health care. Finally the results of prevention and extramural health care are added to compare the results with the data as presented by the OECD on ambulatory health care (to a large extent the summary of Block II: Extramural and Block III: Preventive health care).

Table 12.6
Bilateral Comparison Summary on Block III: Preventive health care (% of GDP)

	Bilateral Comparable Package Block III		
	Netherlands	Other country	Difference [1]
Year 1994			
The Netherlands			
Germany (BCP Netherlands–Germany)	0.27	0.36	0.09
Switzerland (BCP Netherlands–Switzerland)	0.25	0.16	–0.09
Belgium (BCP Netherlands–Belgium)	0.27	0.15	–0.12
Year 1995			
The Netherlands			
Denmark (BCP Netherlands–Denmark)	0.29	0.30	0.01
France (BCP Netherlands–France)	0.29	0.21	–0.08
Switzerland (BCP Netherlands–Switzerland)	0.29	0.14	–0.15
Belgium (BCP Netherlands–Belgium)	0.31	0.14	–0.17

[1] Difference in percentagepoints with respect to the Netherlands.

The amounts on prevention expressed in shares of GDP are very small. Germany spent a substantial larger share on preventive health care activities (0.09 percentage point more than the Netherlands). In Denmark almost the same share of GDP was devoted to prevention compared to the Netherlands (0.35 percent and 0.29 percent respectively). All other countries spent less in percentages of GDP on Block III than the Netherlands. One reason for this can be the lack of sufficiently detailed data on the subject both in the Netherlands and in the other participating countries. Many preventive activities are not a main activity of providers of health care, but subsidies and grants or minor activities in the total package of activities supplied by provisions in the field (extramural/ambulatory health care or intramural health care).

The summary of prevention measured in US $ and in ECU per capita is presented here below.

Table 12.7
Bilateral Comparison Summary on Block III: Preventive health care (US $ & ECU per capita)

	Year	Expenditures per capita	
		US $	Ecu
The Netherlands	1995	73	56
Denmark		100	76
The Netherlands	1994	58	49
Germany		91	77
The Netherlands	1995	73	56
France		56	43
The Netherlands	1994	55	47
Switzerland		60	50
The Netherlands	1995	67	52
Switzerland		75	57
The Netherlands	1994	58	49
Belgium		33	28
The Netherlands	1995	73	56
Belgium		37	28

Only Germany (and to a lesser extent Denmark) spent a "substantial" amount per capita more on preventive health care measured in US dollars per capita, than the Netherlands. France on the other hand seems to spend relatively less than the Netherlands. The difference between the Netherlands and Belgium is quite large but Because the amounts spent on prevention are very small and quite a few assumptions had to made, the relevance of the comparisons is questionable.

Finally the results of the bilateral comparison are compared to the data presented by the OECD on ambulatory care. Therefore the results of the Bilateral Comparisons on extramural health care and prevention are added to one total.

Table 12.8
Bilateral Comparison Summary on Block II + Block III health care (% of GDP)

	OECD Ambulatory care		Bilateral Comparable Package Block II + Block III		
		Difference [1]	Nether-lands	Other country	Difference [1]
Year 1994					
The Netherlands	2.51				
Germany (BCP Netherlands–Germany)	3.06	0.49	2.19	3.65	1.46
Switzerland (BCP Netherlands–Switzerland)	3.60	1.09	2.09	2.88	0.79
Belgium (BCP Netherlands–Belgium)	2.97	0.46	2.18	2.04	–0.14
Year 1995					
The Netherlands	2.47				
Denmark (BCP Netherlands–Denmark)	1.20	–1.27	2.14	1.92	–0.28
France (BCP Netherlands–France)			1.79	2.89	1.10
Switzerland (BCP Netherlands–Switzerland)	3.67	1.2	2.06	2.98	0.92
Belgium (BCP Netherlands–Belgium)	3.02	0.55	2.16	2.17	0.01

[1] Difference in percentagepoints with respect to the Netherlands.

In the chapter on Block II we already mentioned that the OECD Health Data Bank 1997 did not present any data for France on ambulatory health care. So France is left out in the comparison of the OECD data. All countries seem to spend around 3 percent of their GDP on ambulatory health. Only Denmark spent a lot less with only 1.2 percent of their GDP devoted to ambulatory health care.

As could be expected the influence of preventive expenditures on the share of GDP is so small that the difference with respect to the same table in this paragraph on Block II: Extramural health care without prevention is not substantially changed.

Still only Germany and to a lesser extent France and Switzerland spent substantially more on extramural health care and prevention than all others. Only Denmark – followed by Belgium – spent relatively less on extramural health care and prevention than the Netherlands and all other countries.

Note

[1] Health protection: nutritional surveillance, drinking water surveillance, environmental hygiene/surveillance.
Health promotion: health education and information, fight against smoking, fight against alocohol & drugs abuse, prevention of accidents.

13. Bilateral Comparable Package Block IV: Medical goods

13.1 Introduction

Health care goods or medical goods in this project are composed of pharmaceuticals and therapeutic appliances. In the questionnaires on phase II a list of providers was included both for the supply of pharmaceuticals and the supply of therapeutic appliances. In the questionnaire of phase I another composition of these two categories was asked for; among which by kind of goods supplied.

13.2 Supply of pharmaceuticals

Pharmaceuticals can be supplied by pharmacists, general practitioners and specialists, druggists and in some cases by all kinds of other shops (other suppliers). Denmark supplied no division. It is assumed that the amount listed is the total of the expenditure on pharmaceuticals, and that all possible out of pocket expenditures are included.

In Germany almost all the lines of suppliers are filled. The data on druggists are included in the data on pharmacists; data on specialists supplying pharmaceuticals are included in the expenditures of hospitals.

In France all pharmaceuticals supplied are part of the Health Accounts but no specification by category of supplier is given. Pharmaceuticals supplied by hospitals are not included. All non-hospital pharmaceuticals are supplied by pharmacists.

In the Netherlands the data on pharmaceuticals include all categories of suppliers. No division is possible. The data include the expenditures on wound dressings as well, bought either in the pharmacy, drugstore or any other provider of these articles.

Looking at the information and the data supplied by the participants it might be possible that in some countries non-medicine type of pharmaceutical products (e.g. sticking plaster and other kinds of wound dressings) are not included because these expenditures are not included in the health accounts. It might also be possible that some or all out of pocket expenditures are not included for that same reason.

13.3 Supply of therapeutic appliances

according to the questionnaire Therapeutic appliances can be supplied by dental prosthetists, dental technicians, prothetist shops, orthopaedic shoemakers and shops, optician shops, hearing aid shops and a category of (non specified) other suppliers.

Denmark supplied no division by supplier. It is assumed that the total amount supplied consists of the total expenditure on these articles (including out of pocket expenditures).

Germany supplied almost all the categories as requested. Dental technicians expenditures are included in dental prosthetics expenditures and orthopaedic shoemakers expenditures are included in the expenditures of orthopaedic shops. In the category other suppliers Germany provides data on dentists as suppliers of therapeutic appliances.

In France all expenditures on therapeutic appliances are included in the Health Accounts, but only opticals were supplied separately.

Switzerland supplied no data on therapeutic appliances. According to the data delivery these expenditures are included in the expenditures of the Other ambulatory care services (without SPITEX).

No division by supplier is possible for the Netherlands, but all (calculated) out of pocket expenditures are included.

A remark on the dental prosthetics is necessary. In Denmark and Germany these data are included in the therapeutic appliances. Germany supplied separate data on this category of supplier. In the Netherlands, France and Switzerland dental prosthetics and dental technicians are included in the expenditures on Dental practices.

For all participants it is assumed that the expenditures on therapeutic appliances supplied by hospitals are included in the expenditures of these hospitals.

Below the details in the bilateral comparisons in the field of medical goods are supplied for all participants.

13.4 *Bilateral Comparisons*

13.4.1 The Netherlands–Denmark

In Denmark Dental appliances are included in the total of Therapeutic appliances. For the Bilateral Comparison these data have to be calculated either for the Netherlands or for Denmark. It was decided to calculate an amount for Denmark for Dental appliances. This amount was deducted from the Therapeutic appliances and added to the Dental expenditures in extramural health care.

Table 13.1
Results of the Bilateral Comparison Block IV: the Netherlands–Denmark, 1995

	Netherlands	Denmark
	1995	1995
Health care goods(OECD)		
Pharmaceuticals:		
Expenditures per capita (US $)	241	242
Expenditures in % of GDP	0.95	0.73
Therapeutic appliances:		
Expenditures per capita (US $)	67	80
Expenditures in % of GDP	0.26	0.24
Total medical goods:		
Expenditures per capita (US $)	308	322
Expenditures in % of GDP	1.21	0.97
BCP expenditures on Block IV: Medical goods		
Pharmaceuticals:		
Expenditures in US $ (x 1 million)	3,820	1,263
Expenditures in ECU (x 1 million)	2,929	965
Expenditures per capita (US $)	247	242
Therapeutic appliances:		
Expenditures in US $ (x 1 million)	1,034	290
Expenditures in ECU (x 1 million)	792	222
Expenditures per capita (US $)	67	56
Total medical goods:		
Expenditures in US $ (x 1 million)	4,854	1,553
Expenditures in ECU (x 1 million)	3,721	1,186
Expenditures per capita (US $)	314	297
Expenditures per capita (ECU)	240	227
Expenditures in % of GDP	1.23	0.90

The differences between Denmark and the Netherlands are very small in the data presented by the OECD. According to the OECD Denmark spends $ 14 more per capita than the Netherlands caused by a slightly higher expenditure on Therapeutic appliances.

In the Bilateral Package however Denmark spends $ 2,557 million less than the Netherlands on pharmaceuticals and $ 724 million less on therapeutic appliances. This results in a per capita difference of $ 5 on pharmaceuticals and $ 11 on therapeutic appliances that in Denmark is spent less than the Netherlands.

The explanation of this difference between the data in the OECD health data bank and the data supplied for the project is completely clear. Denmark lists the expenditures of dental appliances as Therapeutic appliances; for the project these expenditures are transferred to Block II in the category of Dentist practices.

13.4.2 *The Netherlands–Germany*

In the Netherlands the Dental appliances are a part of the expenditures of Dentist practices. In Germany separate amounts are provided for Dental appliances and dentures in the total of Therapeutic appliances. To make a Bilateral Comparable Package the amount supplied by Germany is deducted from the Therapeutic appliances and added to the expenditures of Dental practices in the field of out-patient health care.

Table 13.2
Results of the Bilateral Comparison Block IV: the Netherlands–Germany, 1994

	Netherlands	Germany
	1994	1994
Health care goods(OECD)		
Pharmaceuticals:		
Expenditures per capita (US $)	206	310
Expenditures in % of GDP	0.94	1.23
Therapeutic appliances:		
Expenditures per capita (US $)	53	152
Expenditures in % of GDP	0.24	0.6
Total medical goods:		
Expenditures per capita (US $)	259	462
Expenditures in % of GDP	1.18	1.83
BCP expenditures on Block IV: Medical goods		
Pharmaceuticals:		
Expenditures in US $ (x 1 million)	3,182	29,408
Expenditures in ECU (x 1 million)	2,681	24,813
Expenditures per capita (US $)	207	361
Therapeutic appliances:		
Expenditures in US $ (x 1 million)	808	5,838
Expenditures in ECU (x 1 million)	681	4,921
Expenditures per capita (US $)	53	72
Total medical goods:		
Expenditures in US $ (x 1 million)	3,991	35,246
Expenditures in ECU (x 1 million)	3,363	29,739
Expenditures per capita (US $)	259	433
Expenditures per capita (ECU)	219	365
Expenditures in % of GDP	1.18	1.72

Germany $ 104 spent more on pharmaceuticals and $ 99 more on therapeutic appliances than the Netherlands according to the OECD data, or 0.65 percentage points of GDP higher in Germany.

In the bilateral comparison the difference is smaller. In total $ 174 Germany spent more on medical goods, caused by the fact that dental appliances and dentures are included in Dental expenditures and not in the therapeutic appliances. The share in GDP for Germany diminishes to 1.72 %, which is 0.54 percentage point higher than in the Netherlands.

13.4.3 *The Netherlands–France*

In France pharmaceuticals are supplied only by pharmacists. The data from France and the Netherlands are presented below.

Table 13.3
Results of the Bilateral Comparison Block IV: the Netherlands–France, 1995

	Netherlands	France
	1995	1995
Health care goods(OECD)		
Pharmaceuticals:		
Expenditures per capita (US $)	241	436
Expenditures in % of GDP	0.95	1.65
Therapeutic appliances:		
Expenditures per capita (US $)	67	64
Expenditures in % of GDP	0.26	0.24
Total medical goods:		
Expenditures per capita (US $)	308	500
Expenditures in % of GDP	1.21	1.89
BCP expenditures on Block IV: Medical goods		
Pharmaceuticals:		
Expenditures in US $ (x 1 million)	3,820	25,716
Expenditures in ECU (x 1 million)	2,929	19,652
Expenditures per capita (US $)	247	443
Therapeutic appliances:		
Expenditures in US $ (x 1 million)	1,034	3,696
Expenditures in ECU (x 1 million)	792	2,825
Expenditures per capita (US $)	67	64
Total medical goods:		
Expenditures in US $ (x 1 million)	4,854	29,413
Expenditures in ECU (x 1 million)	3,781	22,476
Expenditures per capita (US $)	314	506
Expenditures per capita (ECU)	240	387
Expenditures in % of GDP	1.23	1.74

France the expenditures on pharmaceuticals are the highest of all participating countries in the project. Almost $ 200 per capita more is spent on pharmaceuticals than the Netherlands, according to OECD data; on therapeutic appliances the difference is just $ 3 (more in the Netherlands). Measured as percentages of GDP in France 0.68 percentage points is spent more on medical goods. The probable cause is that in France pharmaceuticals are prescribed more easily and in greater quantities, than in the Netherlands.

In the Bilateral Comparison the difference is smaller; France spent $ 192 per capita more on Medical goods than the Netherlands, caused by higher expenditures on pharmaceuticals.

13.4.4 The Netherlands–Switzerland

No additions and deductions are necessary for the Bilateral Comparison of the Netherlands - Switzerland. The only remark that can be made is that the expenditures

Table 13.4
Results of the Bilateral Comparison Block IV: the Netherlands–Switzerland, 1994, 1995

	Netherlands		Switzerland	
	1994	1995	1994	1995
Health care goods(OECD)				
Pharmaceuticals:				
Expenditures per capita (US $)	206	241	264	320
Expenditures in % of GDP	0.94	0.95	0.72	0.75
Therapeutic appliances:				
Expenditures per capita (US $)	53	67		
Expenditures in % of GDP	0.24	0.26		
Total medical goods:				
Expenditures per capita (US $)	259	308	264	320
Expenditures in % of GDP	1.18	1.21	0.72	0.75
BCP expenditures on Block IV: Medical goods				
Pharmaceuticals:				
Expenditures in US $ (x 1 million)	3,182	3,820	2,381	2,931
Expenditures in ECU (x 1 million)	2,681	2,929	2,014	2,232
Expenditures per capita (US $)	207	247	338	409
Therapeutic appliances:				
Expenditures in US $ (x 1 million)	808	1,034	370	478
Expenditures in ECU (x 1 million)	681	792	313	366
Expenditures per capita (US $)	53	67	53	67
Total medical goods:				
Expenditures in US $ (x 1 million)	3,991	4,854	2,751	3,410
Expenditures in ECU (x 1 million)	3,363	3,721	2,326	2,596
Expenditures per capita (US $)	259	314	391	476
Expenditures per capita (ECU)	219	240	331	362
Expenditures in % of GDP	1.18	1.23	1.07	1.11

on therapeutic appliances of Switzerland were included in the Other ambulatory health care services (without SPITEX). For comparability reasons an amount for the expenditures on therapeutic appliances was calculated and transferred from Block II: Extramural health care to Block IV: Medical goods.

The results of the Bilateral Comparison for 1994 and 1995 is presented in table 13.4 (page 174).

According to the OECD Switzerland spent $ 58 more in 1994 and $ 59 more in 1995 on pharmaceuticals than the Netherlands. Switzerland supplies no data on therapeutic appliances in the OECD Health Data Bank, because these suppliers are not distinguished as a separate category in the Swiss Health Accounts.

In the Bilateral Comparison the differences between the total expenditures on Medical goods in Switzerland and the Netherlands are around $ 140 per capita ($ 132 in 1994 and $ 164 in 1995), resulting in a difference in percentages of GDP of 0.10 percentage point in 1994 and 0.12 in 1995.

13.4.5 The Netherlands–Belgium

Belgium supplied data for both 1994 and 1995 on medical goods. On the subject on pharmaceuticals no distinction in sources of providers of pharmaceuticals was given.

Table 13.5
Results of the Bilateral Comparison Block IV: the Netherlands–Belgium, 1994, 1995

	Netherlands		Belgium	
	1994	1995	1994	1995
Health care goods(OECD)				
Pharmaceuticals:				
Expenditures per capita (US $)	206	241	319	384
Expenditures in % of GDP	0.94	0.95	1.41	1.45
Therapeutic appliances:				
Expenditures per capita (US $)	53	67	39	50
Expenditures in % of GDP	0.24	0.26	0.17	0.19
Total medical goods:				
Expenditures per capita (US $)	259	308	358	434
Expenditures in % of GDP	1.18	1.21	1.58	1.64
BCP expenditures on Block IV: Medical goods				
Total medical goods:				
Expenditures in US $ (x 1 million)	3,991	4,854	3,642	4,371
Expenditures in ECU (x 1 million)	3,363	3,721	3,072	3,342
Expenditures per capita (US $)	259	314	360	432
Expenditures per capita (ECU)	219	240	304	330
Expenditures in % of GDP	1.18	1.23	1.59	1.62

Some distinction in suppliers was presented in the therapeutic appliances. The data on medical goods supplied by the OECD and resulting from the Bilateral Comparisons are presented in table 13.5 as well (page 175).

According to the OECD $ 103 per capita is spent more on pharmaceuticals in 1994 and $ 143 in 1995 in Belgium than in the Netherlands. The difference in spending between the Netherlands and Belgium in the therapeutic appliances shows the opposite picture. Belgium spends $ 14 per capita less in 1994 and $ 17 in 1995

On the total of medical goods $ 99 more is spent per capita in Belgium in 1994 than in the Netherlands and $ 126 in 1995.

Because Belgium supplied no division of the Additional payments over the distinct categories (pharmaceuticals and therapeutic appliances) it is not possible to compare these two categories separately for the two countries, only the total of the medical goods can be compared.

13.5 *Summary on the bilateral comparison for medical goods*

A summary on the results of the five bilateral comparisons is given in this last paragraph on medical goods.

Table 13.6
Bilateral Comparison Summary on Block IV: Medical goods (% of GDP)

	OECD Medical goods		Bilateral Comparable Package Block IV		
		Difference [1]	Nether-lands	Other country	Difference [1]
Year 1994					
The Netherlands	1.18				
Germany (BCP Netherlands–Germany)	1.83	0.65	1.18	1.72	0.54
Belgium (BCP Netherlands–Belgium)	1.58	–0.40	1.18	1.59	0.41
The Netherlands	0.94 [2]				
Switzerland (BCP Netherlands–Switzerland)	0.72 [2]	–0.22	1.18	1.07	–0.11
Year 1995					
The Netherlands	1.21				
Denmark (BCP Netherlands–Denmark)	0.97	–0.24	1.23	0.9	–0.33
France (BCP Netherlands–France)	1.89	0.68	1.23	1.74	0.51
Belgium (BCP Netherlands–Belgium)	1.64	–0.43	1.23	1.62	0.39
The Netherlands	0.95 [2]				
Switzerland (BCP Netherlands–Switzerland)	0.75 [2]	0.20	1.23	1.11	–0.12

[1] Difference in percentagepoints with respect to the Netherlands.
[2] Only pharmaceuticals; no expenditures on therapeutic appliances included.

The percentage shares of GDP on OECD data for the comparison the Netherlands–Switzerland relate only to the pharmaceutical expenditures becaue in the OECD Health data bank the expenditures on therapeutic appliances for Switzerland are included in ambulatory health care. In the bilateral comparable packages however a calculation for the expenditures on therapeutic appliances is made and transferred from Block II to Block IV.

In the Comparable Packages for all participants (except Denmark) the differences with the Netherlands measured in percentages of GDP are smaller than in the data presented by the OECD. For Denmark the difference with the Netherlands increases from –0.24 (OECD) to –0.35 percentage point (BCP data).

It comes as no surprise that, the share of GDP spent on Medical goods is larger in Germany and France, taking the low consumption in the Netherlands into consideration.

Below the summary of the data on the Bilateral Comparable Packages is presented calculated in US dollars and ECU per capita.

Table 13.7
Bilateral Comparison Summary on Block IV: Medical goods (US $ & ECU per capita)

	Year	Expenditures per capita	
		US $	Ecu
The Netherlands	1995	314	240
Denmark		293	224
The Netherlands	1994	259	219
Germany		433	365
The Netherlands	1995	314	240
France		506	387
The Netherlands	1994	259	219
Switzerland		391	331
The Netherlands	1995	314	240
Switzerland		476	362
The Netherlands	1994	259	219
Belgium		360	304
The Netherlands	1995	314	240
Belgium		432	330

Measured in US $ per capita the differences are more pronounced. Only the expenditures per capita in Denmark and the Netherlands are almost equal. Denmark spends $ 21 per capita less. France spent $ 192 more on Medical goods, Germany $ 174.

The results of the Netherlands and Switzerland show that $ 132 per capita more was consumed on Medical goods in 1994 and $ 162 in 1995 in Switzerland. It must be noted however that the amount on Therapeutic appliances in the total expenditures on Medical goods for Switzerland is calculated and not supplied by the Swiss Statistical Office.

Belgium also generated more expenditures per capita in the medical goods than the Netherlands. In 1994 Belgium spent $ 101 per capita more and in 1995 $ 122 per capita more than the Netherlands.

14. Attempted Bilateral Comparable Package Block V: Other services

14.1 Introduction

Information on the category of Other services is limited to the expenditures concerning Research & Development, Education & Training and finally Administration.

In almost all Health Accounts the Administration is included as part of the system. Administration is necessary to keep the system running and to implement and check policy measures.

Most of the time Research & Development in the field of health care and Education & Training of health care personnel are not included in the Health Accounts. Because these two categories are connected to health care it was decided to include them in the area of inquiry.

In this chapter we first present the definitions as supplied by the OECD on the area of R&D, Education and Administration, followed by the peculiarities of the Dutch system. Finally the attempted bilateral comparisons and their results in the fields of R&D, Education & Training and Administration will be presented.

14.2 Definitions

The "definitions" presented below are descriptions based on the OECD Health data bank. These descriptions are part of the 1996 edition. In the 1997 edition some minor changes and additions to these descriptive definitions were made but these did not change the essence or meaning of the described subject.

14.2.1 *Research & Development*

Research and Development in the OECD data files is divided in a part on biomedical and a part on pharmaceutical R&D.

Biomedical research comprises the study of specific diseases, including the treatment thereof and rehabilitation; the design of methods, drugs and devices used in the aforementioned process; and finally the scientific investigations in this field leading to new methods, procedures, solutions, etc.

Pharmaceutical research comprises all activities carried out in the enterprise sector.

14.2.2 *Education & Training*

Numbers of students enrolled in paramedical schools, undergraduate schools in medical / biomedical departments and graduate schools in medical / biomedical departments.

It would also include health education reported by local and central authorities for the training of health workers.

Complete expenditures would include universities and other training institutions. Salaries of medical interns, nurse trainees are included in the expenditures of the institutions, not as training expenditures.

14.2.3 *Administration*

Expenditures by private insurers and by central and local authorities including health insurance boards and health boards delivering medical care for planning, management, regulation, fund collecting, handling of claims of the delivery system and other administrative bodies.

Administrative costs born by the providers (such as patient records and hospital management) are not included in general administration.

14.3 *Preliminary remarks*

14.3.1 *Concerning Research & Development (R&D)*

Concerning Research & Development (R&D) two approaches are possible:

- Concentrating on the R&D produced in (all sectors of) the economy on behalf of the health care sector.
- Limiting the R&D to the expenditures of health care providers.

Whatever approach is followed it has to be noted that expenditures in the R&D area are almost always intermediate expenditures in the complete production process (at least of enterprises). In the end the costs of R&D are incorporated in the prices charged for the products sold. The expenditures enter the Health Accounts through these products. Including the expenditures on R&D would lead to a partial double count in the health care expenditures.

14.3.2 *Concerning Training & Education:*

Training & Education concerning health and health care should be limited to the activities in the health care field. This means that only the medical departments of the universities should be included and of course all the educational programs of all institutes educating and training of health care professionals.

The expenditures on Education & Training pose a problem similar to the problem described in the area of R&D. Expenditures in the area of Education can be seen as an investment in human capital. Like investments, outlays are (in a number of cases) excluded from the economic/expenditure accounts of the sector, it would be justified to keep investment in human capital outside the health accounts as well. Depreciation and interest payments are included in the expenditures for the use of investments. For the use of this human capital (a part of) the wage payments can be seen as an equivalent to depreciation, the payment for the use of the capital invested.

14.3.3 *The Netherlands* [1)]

In the Netherlands only the Administration expenditures are part of the health care system and the Health Accounts. The other two activities in the section of Other services, Research & Development and Education & Training, are not part of the Health Accounts.

However data on these two activities were collected. As can be seen in the preliminary remarks some problems were encountered. First of all it had to be decided what approach would yield the best solution in R&D outlays. It was decided to include the R&D focused at the health care sector.

The Netherlands has a survey on R&D expenditures exists. The results of this inquiry were used for the calculation on R&D in health care. Exported and imported R&D was not taken into account. It is possible to make a distinction in enterprises, research institutes and universities. Unfortunately it is not possible to separate R&D in pharmaceutical and biomedical R&D.

In enterprises and research institutes the calculations on expenditures on R&D for health were based on the amount of labour years employed in the medical/ pharmaceutical departments (health sector) relative to the total labour force in the R&D departments.

For the universities the R&D expenditures had to be limited to the medical departments (medicine, veterinarians and dentist). The calculated amount of expenditures was based on the amount of labour in these faculties in relation to total employment in universities. The R&D expenditures of the university faculty of pharmacy are added.

Comparable problems occurred In the area of Education & Training. Financial accounts are available only for universities. A division of the universities in three sectors (health, R&D and education) is available in labour terms. The expenditures on education were based on the number of persons employed in these three sectors.

For all other types of education institutes the financial accounts comprise much more than the education of health care workers. A division of the expenditures was made based on the number of students enrolled in the different areas.

14.4 *Attempted Bilateral comparisons*

Contrary to the other bilateral comparisons (Block I: Intramural, Block II: Extramural, Block III: Prevention and Block IV: Medical goods) in this Bilateral Comparison all three subjects (R&D, Education & Training and Administration) will be presented separately.

In the OECD Health data bank (1997) no expenditure data is available on Education & Training, so a comparison on this area is impossible. On the other two areas (R&D and Administration) for some countries data are presented. As soon as OECD data are available, a comparison with the OECD data will be made.

14.4.1 *The Netherlands–Denmark*

14.4.1.1 *Research & Development*

The data presented by Denmark are for the year 1993, instead of 1995. R&D is performed throughout the economy but only the expenditures on R&D of the universities are included. Special research centres and enterprises are not included. Finally no separation is possible between the two R&D fields.

14.4.1.2 *Administration*

Administrative expenditures in Denmark include the expenditures of local authorities and private insurers next to the expenditures of the central government. Only a few private insurers exist in Denmark. The expenditures attributed to these insurers are a rough estimate and calculation by the Danish participants. Health insurance funds are non-existent in Denmark, so no expenditures in this category are included.
In the Bilateral Comparison it is assumed that the expenditures of the health insurance funds are included in the Danish data of the central and local government.

No meaningful comparison of the OECD data and the data supplied for the bilateral comparison can be made, because only the data on Administration for the Netherlands is supplied in the Health data bank.

Looking at the data supplied in the Bilateral Comparison, the Netherlands and Denmark spend about the same amount on Education & Training ($30 per capita and 0.1 percent of GDP). In R&D Denmark spends almost 70 percent per capita more than the Netherlands. Even on R&D and Education & Training taken together Denmark spends considerably more per capita. It might be questioned if the area under consideration (R&D) has the same meaning in both countries.

In the field of administrative expenditures Denmark spends remarkably little, just over 25 percent of the amount spent in the Netherlands. It is questionable that Administration means the same in both countries.

Table 14.1
Results of the attempted Bilateral Comparison Block V: the Netherlands–Denmark, 1995

	Netherlands 1995			Denmark 1995		
	R&D [1]	E&T [2]	Administration	R&D [1]	E&T [2]	Administration
OECD:						
Expenditures per capita (US $)			100			
Expenditures in % of GDP			0.39			
Attempted BCP expenditures on Block V: Other services						
Expenditures in US $ (x 1 million)	1,072	397	1,489	615	155	124
Expenditures per capita (US $)	69	26	96	118	30	24
Expenditures in % of GDP	0.27	0.10	0.38	0.35	0.09	0.07
		R&D + E&T			*R&D + E&T*	
Expenditures in US $ (x 1 million)		1,442			770	
Expenditures per capita (US $)		95			148	
Expenditures in % of GDP		0.37			0.44	

1) R&D: Research & Development in health care.
2) E&T: Education & Training of health care personnel.

In theory the expenditures in the area R&D by universities are comparable between Denmark and the Netherlands. In the Netherlands 0.17 percent of GDP is spent on R&D by universities. In Denmark this percentage is 0.07, less than half the share of the Netherlands.

14.4.2 *The Netherlands–Germany*

14.4.2.1 Research & Development

R&D in Germany is part of the Health Accounts. In Germany R&D is performed by universities, enterprises and specialised institutions (the so-called blue list of non profit institutions). No division of R&D in pharmaceutical and biomedical R&D is possible. The expenditures presented by Germany are limited to the specialised non profit organisations and the universities. The amounts spent in the private business sector are not known.

14.4.2.2 Education & Training

Education & Training in universities is not a part of the Health Accounts, the education of the nurses and the paramedical professions is included in the Health Accounts. No data are supplied for the education in universities.

14.4.2.3 Administration

All categories listed in the questionnaire on administration are part of the German administrative expenditures. From 1995 onward it is planned to single out the administrative expenditures of the health care providers.

Table 14.2
Results of the attempted Bilateral Comparison Block V: the Netherlands–Germany, 1994

	Netherlands 1994			Germany 1994		
	R&D [1]	E&T [2]	Administration	R&D [1]	E&T [2]	Administration
OECD:						
Expenditures per capita (US $)			87			172
Expenditures in % of GDP			0.40			0.68
Attempted BCP expenditures on Block V: Other services						
Expenditures in US $ (x 1 million)	910	343	1,277	376	4,677	4,420
Expenditures per capita (US $)	59	22	83	5	57	54
Expenditures in % of GDP	0.27	0.10	0.38	0.02	0.23	0.22

[1] R&D: Research & Development in health care.
[2] E&T: Education & Training of health care personnel.

According to the OECD data bank Germany spent about double the amount per capita on Administration compared to the Netherlands. It is obvious that in this context Administration does not mean the same as in the Bilateral Comparison. In the Bilateral Comparison Administration expenditures of Germany are 30 percent less than the amount supplied to the OECD. Looking at the contents of the field as supplied for the project, this data seems better in line with the Dutch data on Administration.

The data on R&D are not comparable between Germany and the Netherlands, because the whole private business sector in missing in Germany.

The data on education are not comparable either (lacking universities). In view of this remark it is even more astonishing that in Germany $35 per capita is spent more on Education & Training of health care workers. Expressed as a percentage of GDP Germany spent twice as much on Education and Training as the Netherlands did.

The expenditures on R&D by universities and specialised research institutes might be comparable between Germany and the Netherlands. The data however do not comply with this statement. In Germany just 0.02 percent of GDP is spent in these categories. In the Netherlands 0.19 percent of GDP is spent on R&D in universities and specialised institutes.

14.4.3 *The Netherlands–France*

14.4.3.1 Research & Development

Like in the other countries mentioned so far France has no separation of the R&D in pharmaceutical and biomedical. Like in the Netherlands R&D is performed in universities, enterprises and specialised research centres. One amount is supplied for the total of the expenditures in this area.

14.4.3.2 Education & Training

Education & Training on the medical field in France is supplied by universities and specialised schools. The expenditures cannot be divided in these two providers of education

14.4.3.3 Administration

Administration is supplied by government bodies, health insurance funds and private insurers. On all these subjects data were supplied.

Table 14.3
Results of the attempted Bilateral Comparison: the Netherlands–France, 1995

	Netherlands 1995			France 1995		
	R&D [1]	E&T [2]	Administration	R&D [1]	E&T [2]	Administration
OECD:						
Expenditures per capita (US $)			100			42
Expenditures in % of GDP			0.39			0.16
Attempted BCP expenditures on Block V: Other services						
Expenditures in US $ (x 1 million)	1,072	397	1,489	5,285	651	9,245
Expenditures per capita (US $)	69	26	96	91	11	159
Expenditures in % of GDP	0.27	0.10	0.38	0.34	0.04	0.60
		R&D + E&T			*R&D + E&T*	
Expenditures in US $ (x 1 million)		1,442			5,936	
Expenditures per capita (US $)		95			102	
Expenditures in % of GDP		0.37			0.38	

1) R&D: Research & Development in health care.
2) E&T: Education & Training of health care personnel.

Looking at the administrative expenditures in the OECD Health data and comparing those with the data supplied for the Bilateral Comparison the data show a complete different picture for both countries. In the OECD data France spends $ 60 per capita less; in the attempted BCP France spends $ 63 per capita more. The cause for this apparent difference in the results is that France supplied data on the expenditures of Administration, which are not included in the data supplied to the OECD for the Health Data Bank (notably data of Health Insurance Funds / Boards and on Other administrative agencies).

Both expenditures on R&D and on Education & training should be comparable. In both countries the contents of the areas are the same. So it is probably valid to state that France spent 50 percent more per capita on R&D. For R&D expressed as a percentage of GDP France spends 25 percent more than the Netherlands.

On the other hand education in the Netherlands is twice as expensive per capita compared to France. Expressed in shares of GDP the Netherlands spends 2.5 times more than France.

14.4.4 *The Netherlands–Switzerland*

14.4.4.1 Research & Development

R&D in Switzerland is supplied by universities, enterprises and specialised research centres. Central government plays some part in the R&D on pharmaceuticals. In the data however just the amounts supplied by a specialised fund in Switzerland are included.

14.4.4.2 Education & Training

Like in all other countries Education & Training is provided by universities and special schools. Education & Training is no part of the Health Accounts. The data included the medical departments and the education of nursing and social professions.

14.4.4.3 Administration

Mentioned as administrative bodies are government bodies and health insurance boards. Private insurers, although they exist in Switzerland, are not mentioned. The data supplied by Switzerland contain the data on government bodies and health insurance funds. The data of private insurers are not included. A calculation of the expenditures of private insurers was made in order to get a more comparable picture.

In Switzerland R&D expenditures are financed by a special fund. There are no specified data regarding universities, enterprises and specialised research centres. Therefore the data are not comparable. This is true for both 1994 and 1995.

In the area of education comparability should exist, in view of the descriptions presented in this area. Looking at the data some doubts arise as to the comparability. If comparability exists it would mean that the education of health care workers is four to five times more expensive per capita in Switzerland than in the Netherlands. As a share in GDP it is 0.18 percentage point more expensive in Switzerland (more than double the share of the Netherlands)

Table 14.4
Results of the attempted Bilateral Comparison Block V: the Netherlands-Switzerland, 1994

	Netherlands 1994			Switzerland 1994		
	R&D [1]	E&T [2]	Administration	R&D [1]	E&T [2]	Administration
OECD:						
Expenditures per capita (US $)			87			154
Expenditures in % of GDP			0.40			0.50
Attempted BCP expenditures on Block V: Other services						
Expenditures in US $ (x 1 million)	910	343	1,277	126	792	1,464
Expenditures per capita (US $)	59	22	83	18	104	208
Expenditures in % of GDP	0.27	0.10	0.38	0.05	0.28	0.57

1) R&D: Research & Development in health care.
2) E&T: Education & Training of health care personnel.

Table 14.4 (end)
Results of the attempted Bilateral Comparison Block V: the Netherlands-Switzerland, 1995

	Netherlands 1995			Switzerland 1995		
	R&D [1]	E&T [2]	Administration	R&D [1]	E&T [2]	Administration
OECD:						
Expenditures per capita (US $)			100			165
Expenditures in % of GDP			0.39			0.51
Attempted BCP expenditures on Block V: Other services						
Expenditures in US $ (x 1 million)	1,072	397	1,489	155	818	1,880
Expenditures per capita (US $)	69	26	96	22	114	262
Expenditures in % of GDP	0.27	0.1	0.38	0.05	0.27	0.61

1) R&D: Research & Development in health care.
2) E&T: Education & Training of health care personnel.

Looking at the data supplied for the OECD Health data bank 1997 it can be seen that Switzerland spent almost twice the amount per capita on Administration compared to the Dutch (in 1994). Switzerland like in the majority of all other Blocks spends absolutely the largest amount per capita ($ 154 in 1994 and $ 165 in 1995) on Administration. In the Bilateral Comparison the same picture emerges. Switzerland is the biggest spender also on Administration; the differences with respect to the expenditures of the Netherlands are even larger.

14.4.5 *The Netherlands–Belgium*

Belgium did not supply any information on the subject of R&D and Education & Training, only on administrative outlays, so only a comparison was made in this area. Due to the fact that in the OECD Health data bank there are no data on administrative expenditures no comparison with the OECD is possible.

Table 14.5
Results of the attempted Bilateral Comparsion Block V: the Netherlands-Belgium, 1994, 1995

	Netherlands		Belgium	
	1994	1995	1994	1995
	Administration		Administration	
Attempted BCP expenditures on Block V: Other services				
Expenditures in US $ (x 1 million)	1,277	1,489	658	740
Expenditures per capita (US $)	83	96	65	73
Expenditures in % of GDP	0.38	0.38	0.29	0.28

Comparing the data supplied for the project on international comparability the Netherlands spent one third more on Administration per capita as Belgium, both for 1994 and 1995.

14.5 *Concluding remark*

It is obvious that more information is needed and more data are necessary to create Bilateral Comparable Packages (BCP) and in the end a Common Comparable Package (CCP). Calculations especially on R&D of health care are impossible because no plausible assumptions can be made.

For now more comparable BCP's can not be made, so the construction of a CCP on Other services is not feasible.

14.5.1 *Administration*

Because data are supplied on the subject of administrative expenditures for all participants this topic is included in the construction of the BCP and the CCP. A separate line on Administration is included in the comparisons.
The summary data on the topic of Administration is presented below, first in percentages of GDP and finally in US dollars and in ECU per capita.

Table 14.6
Bilateral Comparison Summary on Administration (% of GDP)

	OECD Administration		Bilateral Comparable Package Block V		
		Difference [1]	Nether-lands	Other country	Difference [1]
Year 1994					
The Netherlands	0.39				
Germany (BCP Netherlands–Germany)	0.68	0.29	0.38	0.22	–0.16
Switzerland (BCP Netherlands–Switzerland)	0.50	0.11	0.38	0.57	0.19
Belgium (BCP Netherlands–Belgium)			0.38	0.29	–0.09
Year 1995					
The Netherlands	0.40				
Denmark (BCP Netherlands–Denmark)	0.16	–0.24	0.38	0.07	–0.31
France (BCP Netherlands–France)			0.38	0.60	0.22
Switzerland (BCP Netherlands–Switzerland)	0.51	0.11	0.38	0.61	0.23
Belgium (BCP Netherlands–Belgium)			0.38	0.28	–0.10

[1] Difference in percentagepoints with respect to the Netherlands.

No data on administrative expenditures are presented for Belgium and Denmark in the OECD Health data bank. For the other countries the figures presented raise some questions on the comparability of the data. Referring to the Netherlands as the key country, Germany spends almost twice and France not even half the amount of the Netherlands. Data for all participants are available in the Bilateral Packages. But still there are large difference. Belgium and Germany spent about 0.10 percentage point less than the Netherlands. On the other hand Switzerland and France spend al lot more (over 0.2 percentage point of GDP).

A comparison of the data from the OECD and the data in the project shows that the contents of the packages cannot be the same. For Germany the package included in the comparison contains fewer provisions than included in the German health care system, and presumably provisions with a high administrative burden. For France on the other hand it seems that a lot of administrative expenditures not included in the French health accounts are included for the project.

In table 14.7 on page 190 the same picture emerges if the data on Administration are calculated in US dollars and in ECU. Although according to the descriptions supplied by the participants all the items mentioned in the questionnaire exist there are large differences between the countries. Denmark spent only ECU 18 per capita on Administration being one quarter of the Dutch expenditures on Administration. Switzerland spent ECU 200 per capita, over 2.5 times more than the Netherlands and eleven times more than Denmark.

Table 14.7
Bilateral Comparison Summary on Administration (US $ & ECU per capita)

	Year	Expenditures per capita	
		US $	Ecu
The Netherlands	1995	96	74
Denmark		24	18
The Netherlands	1994	83	70
Germany		54	46
The Netherlands	1995	96	74
France		159	121
The Netherlands	1994	83	70
Switzerland		208	176
The Netherlands	1995	96	74
Switzerland		226	200
The Netherlands	1994	83	70
Belgium		65	55
The Netherlands	1995	96	74
Belgium		73	54

Note

1) The authors would like to thank Mrs. M.F.C. Freese for the research on the Dutch data section.

15. Input and BCP compared

15.1 Introduction

For all Blocks I through IV Bilateral Comparable Packages were constructed, so it was possible to compare the contents of the BCP Blocks and the input as supplied by the participants.

For all participants the data as supplied for Research & Development and Education & Training in the category Other services were excluded in the addition of the input. The reason is the diversity of the data supplied very detailed for some countries on some subjects and no data or very limited or roughly estimated data on other subjects.

Included however are the data on the administrative outlays of all participants

The results of the Bilateral Comparisons are presented below in relation to the original input as supplied by the participants for Phase II of the project.

Table 15.1
Input and BCP Block I to Block IV & Administration, 1994, 1995 (million US $ & percentage

	Year	Expenditures in US $ (x 1 million)		BCP as % of Input
		Input	BCP	
The Netherlands	1995	34,922	29,768	85
Denmark		13,674	10,722	78
The Netherlands	1994	29,716	28,307	95
Germany		213,764	204,593	96
The Netherlands	1995	34,922	27,768	79
France		153,174	150,921	99
The Netherlands	1994	29,716	29,340	99
Switzerland		24,671	24,791	100
The Netherlands	1995	34,922	34,547	99
Switzerland		29,703	30,125	101
The Netherlands	1994	29,716	27,763	93
Belgium		16,201	17,402	107
The Netherlands	1995	34,922	32,700	94
Belgium		19,368	20,818	107

15.2 The Netherlands–Denmark

In the construction of the first Bilateral Comparison, the Netherlands–Denmark, on balance we used 85 percent of the input for the Netherlands and 78 percent for Denmark.

For the Netherlands the largest provisions not included in the BCP are the Institution for the mentally deficient and the Nursing homes, totalling $ 5,600 million or 16 percent of the input. For Denmark some institutions providing long term care (like Nursing home care, Integrated care schemes and provisions for the disabled) are not included in the BCP. These provisions amount to $ 2,500 million, or 18 percent of the input.

15.3 *The Netherlands–Germany*

For the Netherlands we excluded only the Institutions for mentally deficient ($ 3,300 million). For Germany the situation is more complicated. In the input for 1994 no data are supplied for some specific German features such as the cost of income compensation in case of illness and disability, the cost of occupational and social rehabilitation in case of illness and disability and specific financial support in case of illness. These specific features are not included in the input file of Germany and play no part in the input of Phase II.

Specifically for Germany the Health spas are not included in the BCP amounting to $ 1,300 million.

15.4 *The Netherlands–France*

In the construction of the BCP for the Netherlands–France we excluded the Institutions for the mentally deficient and the Nursing home for the Netherlands (about 16 percent of the input).

For France on the other hand we excluded only a few very small parts of provisions, leaving 99 percent of the input for the BCP.

15.5 *The Netherlands–Switzerland*

In the construction of the BCP for the Netherlands and Switzerland less than 1 percent of the input was left out for both countries, resulting in a BCP containing almost 100 percent of the input in either country.

15.6 *The Netherlands–Belgium*

For the Netherlands we included 93 percent of the input in the BCP with Belgium. Not included are e.g. the mentally deficient ($ 3,300 million) responsible for almost 9 percent.

In the Belgian input file, only the expenditures for the responsibility of the health authorities are included for some provisions. The remainder of these expenditures had to be calculated or estimated before they could be included in the BCP. Together with an estimation of the supplementary insurance these data are responsible for the fact that in Belgium 107 percent of the input is used for the BCP.

15.7 *Summary on the comparison of Input and Bilateral Comparable Package*

Graphs 15.1 and 15.2 show the Bilateral Comparable Packages of the participants in relation to the input as supplied.

In 1994 at least 95 percent of the input was used (in the BCP of the Netherlands and Germany). The maximum used is 107 percent for Belgium. In 1995 the input in relation to the Bilateral Packages ranged from 78 percent for Denmark to again 107 for Belgium.

Graph 15.1 Input and BCP Block I to Block IV & Administration, 1994

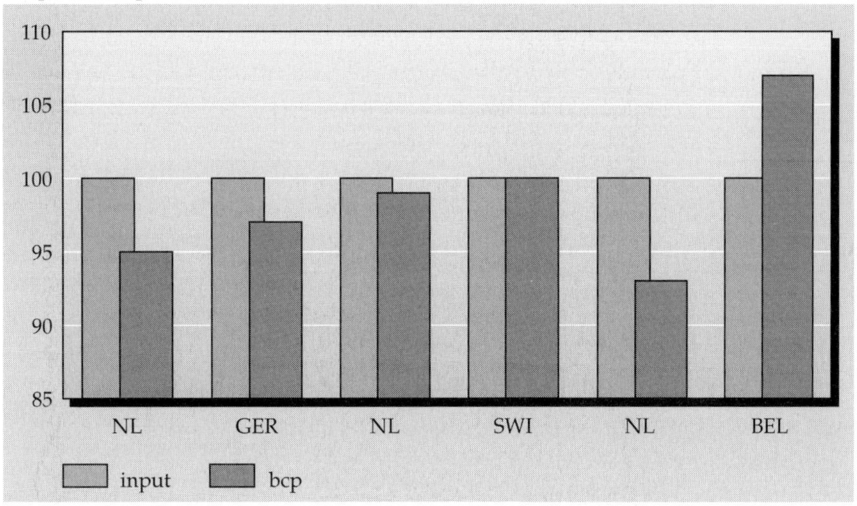

Graph 15.2 Input and BCP Block I to Block IV & Administration, 1995

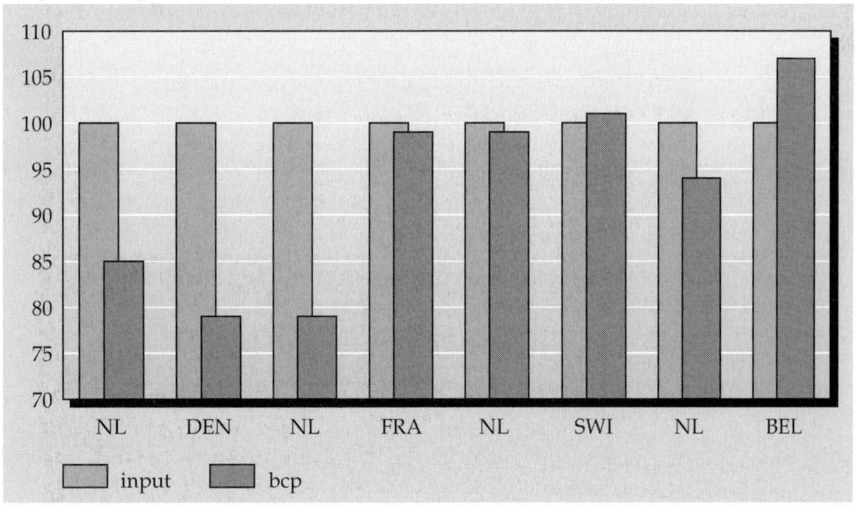

16. Common Comparable Packages: Introduction

This chapter deals with the development of a "Common Comparable Package" (CCP) for the six participating countries, based on the available Bilateral Comparisons.

The CCP consists of provisions selected from the lists of provisions used for the Bilateral Comparisons of the five countries considered. In principle these provisions are counted as part of the health care systems in the participating countries.

As already mentioned in the construction of the BCP in the Netherlands some provisions that were no part of the health accounts on historical grounds are included. These provisions are separately listed (as provisions outside health accounts).

The Common Comparable Package (CCP) is not limited to provisions existing in all participating countries. An extension of participants in the process would almost certainly lead to a diminishing number of provisions in the CCP.

The Common Comparable Package on the other hand does not include all provisions listed as health care in any of the participating countries. An extension of the number of participating countries could (ate least in theory) lead to an continuous expanding of the Common Comparable Package.

So on pragmatic grounds provisions part of Block I: Intramural health care in one country and included in the Block II: Extramural health care sector (e.g. Midwifes practices in the Netherlands) or in the social sector in yet another country (like Nursing homes in Denmark) are enclosed in the CCP. On the other hand some provisions included in health care in some countries (e.g. Day care centres or Institutions for the mentally handicapped) are not considered as health care in other countries and as a consequence deducted and eliminated from the bilateral comparison results.

On analogy to the construction of the CCP for Block I, CCP's for the other Blocks (except Block V: other services) are created.

The results of the five Bilateral Comparisons are the starting point of every chapter in the construction of a Common Comparable Package. To create a CCP for all participants additions and deductions are necessary in terms of provisions and/or activities. In some cases for these additions and deductions calculations and assumptions were necessary A complete list of all provisions added and deducted is presented in the chapters dealing with the various subjects.

In the following chapters the various CCP's are presented, starting with the CCP on Block I: Intramural health care and ending with Block IV: Medical goods

17. Common Comparable Package Block I: Intramural health care: update

17.1 Introduction

In this chapter we present the construction of the Common Comparable Package on Block I: Intramural health care. Like in phase I the starting points are the constructed Bilateral Comparable Packages for all participants. Next provisions will be added and deducted to reach one package of provisions providing activities that are common to all participants.

First the Bilateral Packages will be presented. Next are the calculations needed and assumptions followed by the resulting CCP Block I.

17.2 The Bilateral Comparable Packages

The results of the update on intramural health care as presented below in of Chapter 4 are the starting point in the construction of a CCP on Block I.

Table 17.1
Block I health care expenditures 1994 (Summary of the Bilateral Comparison)

	Nether-lands	Germany	Nether-lands	Switzer-land	Nether-lands	Belgium
	1994		1994		1994	
BCP expenditures on Block I:						
Intramural health care						
Expenditures						
US $ (x 1 million)	15,688	92,286	17,030	13,147	15,158	8,213
Expenditures						
ECU (x 1 million)	13,219	77,866	14,349	11,119	12,772	6,929

Looking at the data on Block I health care presented for the Netherlands it is clear that the contents of Block I is not the same in the five Bilateral Comparisons. In 1994 as well as 1995 different figures on expenditures are presented for the Netherlands. It is also obvious that the contents of Block I is not the same for the other five countries. In the Netherlands some $ 15.1 thousand million is included in the BCP with Belgium in 1994. In the BCP with Switzerland $ 20.0 thousand million (1994) is included for the Netherlands. The difference for the Netherlands for 1994 (comparing the Netherands–Switzerland) is roughly 4,000 million US $. For the Netherlands–Belgium the gap is almost $ 8,000 million. In 1995 to gaps to bridge are of the same order of magnitude.

Table 17.1 (end)
Block I health care expenditures 1995 (Summary of the Bilateral Comparison)

	Nether-lands	Den-mark	Nether-lands	France	Nether-lands	Switzer-land	Nether-lands	Belgium
	1995		1995		1995		1995	
BCP expenditures on Block I: Intramural health care								
Expenditures US $ (x 1 million)	14,986	5,810	14,355	67,732	20,073	15,720	17,855	9,859
Expenditures ECU (x 1 million)	11,489	4,439	11,006	51,758	15,389	11,968	13,689	7,545

To create a common comparable package for all six countries it is necessary to add and subtract provisions.

17.3 *Additions and Deductions*

Like in phase I the following provisions were added, if these provisions were no part of the Bilateral Packages yet. Added are Hospital out patient departments, Treatment of alcoholics and drugs abuse, Other mental health care services, Medical laboratories, Midwifes services, Short term recovery homes, Nursing homes, Institutions for supervised dwelling under medical supervision, 24 Hour care and Integrated care institutions.

Subtracted are the Day centres for the physically disabled, Institutions for the mentally deficient, Homes for the sensorial handicapped, the Occupational and social rehabilitation and the Homes for the elderly.

17.4 *Towards a CCP on Block I: Intramural health care*

All the additions and subtractions mentioned above lead to the following table, presenting a common comparable package for Block I provisions for the six participating countries.

Table 17.2
Towards a CCP on Block I health care, 1994 (US $)

	Nether-lands	Germany	Nether-lands	Switzer-land	Nether-lands	Belgium
	1994		1994		1994	
	US $ (x 1 million)					
BCP Block I	15,688	92,286	17,030	13,147	15,158	8,213
Additions			513	258	559	404
Deductions			1,855	1,280	29	
CCP Block I	15,688	92,286	15,688	1,126	15,688	8,617

Table 17.2 (end)
Towards a CCP on Block I health care, 1995 (US $)

	Nether-lands	Den-mark	Nether-lands	France	Nether-lands	Switzer-land	Nether-lands	Belgium
	1995		1995		1995		1995	
	US $ (x 1 million)							
BCP Block I	14,986	5,800	14,355	67,732	20,073	15,720	17,855	9,859
Additions	3,506	2,399	4,136	15,313	581	312	636	458
Deductions	37		37	1,805	2,200	1,586	37	
CCP Block I	18,454	8,203	18,454	81,241	18,454	14,446	18,454	10,318

The following table presents a summary of the results of the Bilateral Comparisons and the Common Comparable Package in terms of expenditures on Intramural health care as a share of GDP.

Table 17.3
BCP and CCP Block I health care, 1994, 1995 (% of GDP)

	Year	BCP Block I		CCP Block I	
			Difference 1)		Difference 1)
The Netherlands	1995	3.80		4.68	
Denmark		3.35	-0.45	4.74	0.06
The Netherlands	1994	4.66		4.66	
Germany		4.50	-0.76	4.30	-0.76
The Netherlands	1995	3.64		4.68	
France		4.40	0.76	5.28	0.60
The Netherlands	1994	5.06		4.66	
Switzerland		5.10	0.04	4.71	0.05
The Netherlands	1995	5.09		4.68	
Switzerland		5.12	0.03	4.71	0.03
The Netherlands	1994	4.50		4.66	
Belgium		3.58	-0.92	3.76	-0.90
The Netherlands	1995	4.53		4.68	
Belgium		3.66	-0.87	3.84	-0.84

1) Difference in percentagepoints with respect to the Netherlands.

In the Bilateral Packages the shares of the Dutch GDP devoted to health varies from 3.62 percent in the BCP Netherlands–France to 5.09 percent in the BCP Netherlands–Switzerland. Noteworthy is that the share of the Netherlands is high in comparison with all other countries. The Dutch share is low only in comparison with France. An obvious reason for the relatively important position of the Dutch intramural health care is the inclusion of a large segment of the expenditures of self-employed specialists in Block I: Intramural health.

Looking at the results of the constructed CCP the differences between the Netherlands and the other participating countries are smaller than in the BCP. So it seems that the shares spend on Block I expressed in percentages of GDP are more in line throughout the countries. The Netherlands and Switzerland spend 4.7 percent of their GDP on Block I in the CCP on health; Germany 4.4. percent, France 5.7 percent. Belgium is still the country that spent the least on Block I with 3.8 percent of GDP in 1994 and 1995.

The last table in this paragraph shows the data on the CCP measured in US $ and ECU per capita

Table 17.4
CCP on Block I: Intramural health care, 1994, 1995 (US $ and ECU per capita)

	Year	Expenditures per capita	
		US $	Ecu
The Netherlands	1995	1,192	914
Denmark		1,572	1,201
The Netherlands	1994	1,020	859
Germany		1,133	956
The Netherlands	1995	1,192	914
France		1,398	1,068
The Netherlands	1994	1,020	859
Switzerland		1,723	1,457
The Netherlands	1995	1,192	908
Switzerland		2,016	1,535
The Netherlands	1994	1,020	859
Belgium		852	719
The Netherlands	1995	1,192	914
Belgium		1,019	780

The expenditures on the CCP expressed in US $ per capita show that Switzerland spent the largest amount by (still 70 percent more than the Netherlands), followed by Denmark and France. and Germany. Belgium spent least of all participants. Expressed in ECU values the data present an analogous result.

Lastly graph 17.1 gives a graphic representation of the process. At the start of the project (1994) only the OECD shares of in-patient care (indicated by the letter O and a country index) were available. Comparability was believed to be questionable. As a first step Bilateral Comparable Packages were composed; the results of which are indicated by the letters BCP and country indices. Bilateral Comparable Packages are not equivalent to mutual, common comparability between all countries. To reach a more common comparable number, the steps described in this chapter were necessary. The shares of the CCP in GDP are indicated by the letters CCP and a country index.

Graph 17.1 Block I health care: OECD, BCP & CCP compared, 1994, 1995 (% of GDP)

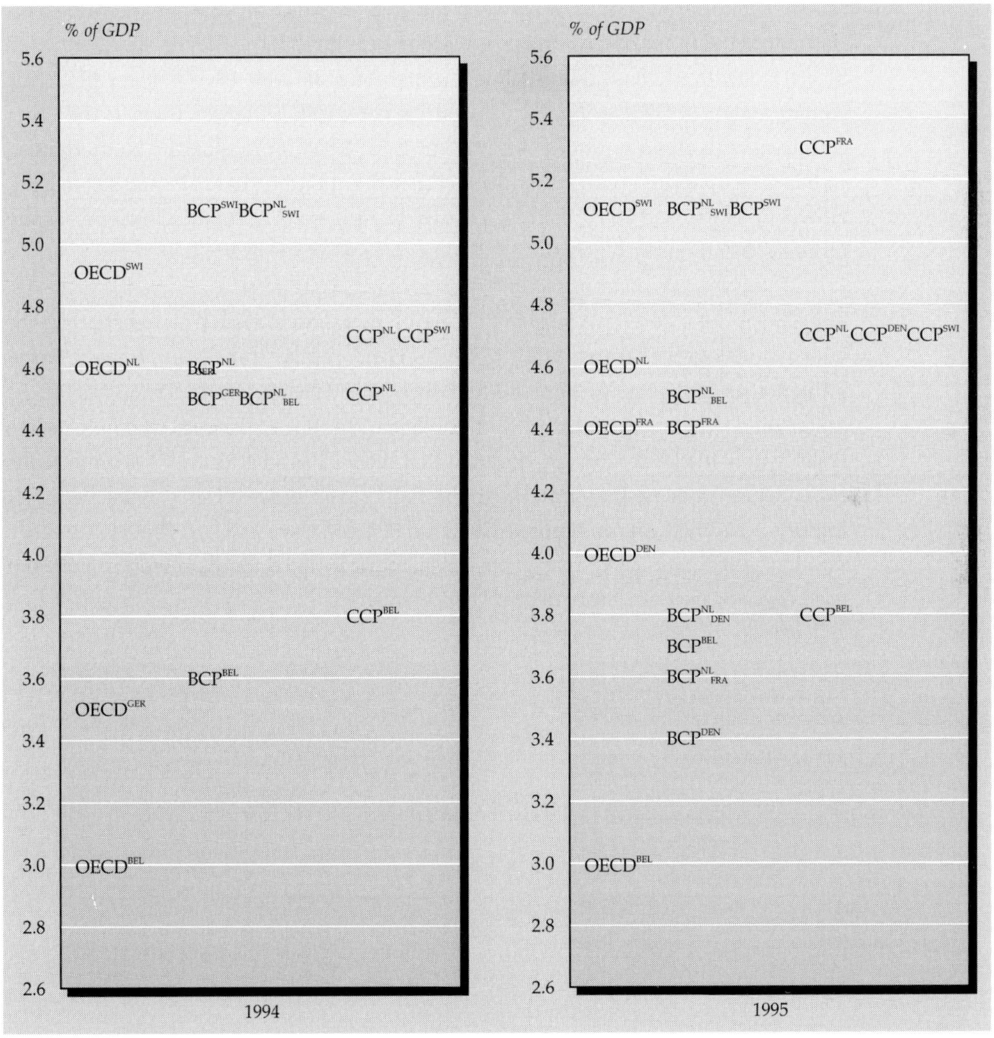

Comparing the OECD shares of in-patient health care in GDP with the shares of the CCP it can be concluded that the shares in the CCP are closer together than those of the OECD, the only exception being France.

17.5 *Concluding remarks*

The differences between the countries are not big in terms of percentages of GDP. In Germany the share of GDP devoted to the CCP on Block I health care is 4.4 percent, relatively low compared to the other countries. Germany is known for its large and important ambulatory health care sector.

France on the contrary has a very large in-patient sector (5.3 percent of GDP). These differences are not reflected in the expenditures on the CCP expressed in US $ per capita. The difference in US $ between the Netherlands and Germany is some $ 87. Compared to France the difference is $ 266 per capita that the French spend more on Block I. Denmark has a high Block I spending as well ($ 366 more than the Netherlands). In Switzerland the spending per capita is larger than in the other countries with an amount of US $ 2,007 in 1995 ($ 819 more than the Netherlands). To a large extent this is caused by the fact that all expenditures are expressed in US $. However, expressed in ECU values the Swiss still spent some ECU 600 per capita more in 1995 than the Dutch.

The US $ is not a good measure in the case of Switzerland with its large share in the international capital transaction. In Switzerland capital transaction have a larger influence on the currency demand and supply and hence the exchange rate of the dollar than the import and export of goods and services. Although the ECU is less volatile than the US dollar, it is doubted that the ECU is a better way to compare the expenditure data in the same year. In time series however it can be of major importance which denominator will be used (US dollars or ECU's). That is the reason that in the comparison of two years (for a country) the data expressed in ECU are used and not the data expressed in US dollars.

18. Common Comparable Package Block II: Extramural health care

18.1 Introduction

In this chapter the construction of the CCP on Block II: Extramural health care is described.

The starting point is the Bilateral Comparable Packages (BCP's) as constructed in chapter 11. Next the provisions to be added from other Blocks are included and finally the deductions from the BCP are introduced. The deductions include the activities and provisions that are transferred to Block I on Intramural health care. The results is a Common Comparable Package.

18.2 The Bilateral Comparable Packages

The starting point BCP Block II: Extramural health care for the six participating countries is presented below.

Table 18.1
Block II health care expenditures 1994 (Summary of the Bilateral Comparison)

	Netherlands	Germany	Netherlands	Switzerland	Netherlands	Belgium
	1994		1994		1994	
BCP expenditures on Block II: Extramural health care						
Expenditures US $ (x 1 million)	6,452	67,350	6,193	7,009	6,444	4,556
Expenditures ECU (x 1 million)	5,437	56,827	5,218	5,927	5,430	3,844

Table 18.1 (end)
Block II health care expenditures 1995 (Summary of the Bilateral Comparison)

	Netherlands	Denmark	Netherlands	France	Netherlands	Switzerland	Netherlands	Belgium
	1995		1995		1995		1995	
BCP expenditures on Block II: Extramural health care								
Expenditures US $ (x 1 million)	7,302	2,805	5,929	41,294	7,087	8,577	7,371	5,470
Expenditures ECU (x 1 million)	5,598	2,143	4,542	31,555	5,435	6,529	5,651	4,186

18.3 *Additions & Deductions*

From the Bilateral Comparable Packages the Psychotherapists, the Institutions providing treatment for alcoholics and drug abusers, the Other ambulatory mental health care institutions, Medical laboratories and Midwifes are excluded and transferred to Block I. These activities are already included in the CCP on Block I.

Just one provision is added: Maternity home care. In all countries except Switzerland this kind of activity is included in the health accounts. In Switzerland this provision is, although existent, is not included in the Health accounts. A calculation for the addition is made.

From the BCP on Block II: Extramural health care the Home help (as distinguished from the activity home/district nursing) is subtracted. The reason is that Home help, although linked to health care in some countries, is basically a social service and not a health care service.

Only in the case of Switzerland the Home help activity poses a problem. Home help and the Home district nurse activity are activities provided by one type of provision. So a separation of these two provisions was made.

18.4 *Towards a CCP on Block II: Extramural health care*

In the table below the results of the transfers to Block I and de additions and deductions are presented.

Table 18.2
Towards a CCP on Block II health care, 1994 (US $)

	Netherlands	Germany	Netherlands	Switzerland	Netherlands	Belgium
	1994		1994		1994	
	US $ (x 1 million)					
BCP Block II	6,452	67,350	6,193	7,009	6,444	4,556
Additions			218	100	8	8
Deductions	1,734	6,602	1,693	566	1,734	820
CCP Block II	4,718	60,749	4,718	6,543	4,718	3,384

As mentioned in the previous chapter on Block I health care the transfers range from $ 111 million in the case of Denmark to $ 6,227 million in case of Germany. For the Netherlands about $ 500 million on average was transferred from Block II to Block I in 1994. Belgium is the exception with a transfer of $ 404 million.

Table 18.2 (end)
Towards a CCP on Block II health care, 1995 (US $)

	Netherlands	Denmark	Netherlands	France	Netherlands	Switzerland	Netherlands	Belgium
	1995		1995		1995		1995	
	US $ (x 1 million)							
BCP Block II	7,302	2,805	5,925	41,294	7,087	8,577	7,371	5,470
Additions					244	113	10	9
Deductions	1,929	707	552	4,378	1,958	714	2,008	1,359
CCP Block II	5,373	2,097	5,373	36,916	5,373	7,976	5,373	4,119

Due to the fact that only a few provisions are additionally deducted, the amounts involved are in the same order of magnitude. For the Netherlands some 1.7 thousand million US $ is deducted in 1994; for Switzerland only 566 million in the same year.

Only for the BCP Netherlands–Switzerland and for the BCP of the Netherlands–Belgium required additions. For the Netherlands and Belgium the additions were close to zero (US $ 8 million in 1994 and $ 9 million in 1995); for the Netherlands and Switzerland the additions amounted to $ 218 and $ 100 million respectively.

For the year 1995 the amounts deducted were on average $ 200 million higher for the Netherlands. The exception being the BCP with France. In this BCP, only $ 552 is deducted for the Netherlands. No additions were necessary for Denmark and France (like for Germany in 1994).

18.5 *The results of the CCP on Block II: Extramural health care*

In this paragraph the results of the CCP for the six countries are described. First (in the table below) the BCP's and the CCP on Block II: Extramural health care expressed in percentages of GDP are compared. Next the CCP measured in US $ and ECU per capita is presented.

Looking at the BCP as a percentage of GDP it is obvious that Block II is small in the Netherlands compared to France, Switzerland and Germany; compared to Denmark it is bigger. The main reason for this pattern can be the treatment of the expenditures of specialists in the Netherlands (some 84% of the Self-employed specialist practices is attributed to Block I: Intramural health care). The explanation for the relative small share of Denmark may be that activities performed in a Block II: Extramural setting in the other countries are delivered by Block I: Intramural institutions in Denmark.

The non-intramural health care sector in Germany is relatively more important. Of course it is still possible that some activities listed as Block II health care in one country are listed as preventive health care in another country and vice versa.

Table 18.3
BCP an CCP on Block II health care, 1994, 1995 (% of GDP)

	Year	BCP Block II		CCP Block II	
			Difference [1]		Difference [1]
The Netherlands	1995	1.85		1.36	
Denmark		1.62	-0.23	1.21	-0.15
The Netherlands	1994	1.92		1.40	
Germany		3.29	1.37	2.96	1.56
The Netherlands	1995	1.50		1.36	
France		2.68	1.18	2.40	1.04
The Netherlands	1994	1.84		1.4	
Switzerland		2.72	0.88	2.54	1.14
The Netherlands	1995	1.80		1.36	
Switzerland		2.80	1.00	2.60	1.24
The Netherlands	1994	1.91		1.40	
Belgium		1.99	0.08	1.47	0.07
The Netherlands	1995	1.87		1.36	
Belgium		2.03	0.16	1.53	0.17

[1] Difference in percentagepoints with respect to the Netherlands.

The CCP on Block II health care shows that the differences between the Netherlands and two other countries are larger (compared to the BCP's), i.e. with Germany and Switzerland. This can only mean that the amount deducted for the Netherlands is relatively more important than in these other two countries, which is likely because of the deduction related to Home help. For Denmark and France the relative difference with to the Netherlands is smaller in the CCP than in the BCP on Block II care.

Table 18.4 (page 207) shows the results measured in US $ and ECU per capita.

Of course the same differences can be seen in the amounts spent on Block II health care per capita as in percentages of GDP. The amount that the Swiss spend on Block II health care is striking; over three times more than the Dutch and even almost 25 percent more than the Germans. Measured in ECU the relative differences are not different from those in US dollars.

Table 18.4
CCP on Block II: Extramural health care, 1994, 1995 (US $ & ECU per capita)

	Year	Expenditures per capita	
		US $	Ecu
The Netherlands	1995	347	266
Denmark		402	307
The Netherlands	1994	307	258
Germany		746	630
The Netherlands	1995	347	266
France		635	486
The Netherlands	1994	307	258
Switzerland		930	786
The Netherlands	1995	347	266
Switzerland		1,113	847
The Netherlands	1994	307	256
Belgium		335	282
The Netherlands	1995	347	266
Belgium		407	311

19. Common Comparable Package Block III: Prevention

19.1 Introduction

This chapter describes the way towards a Common Comparable Package for Block III on prevention. Starting with the BCP's on prevention, first the provisions to be included in the Block I CCP will be deducted. This is followed by the additions and deductions necessary to construct a CCP on preventive health care are presented.

19.2 The Bilateral Comparable Packages

he starting point of this part of this paragraph, the Bilateral Packages on Block III is presented below.

Table 19.1
Block III health care expenditures 1994 (Summary of the Bilateral Comparison)

	Netherlands	Germany	Netherlands	Switzerland	Netherlands	Belgium
	1994		1994		1994	
BCP expenditures on Block III: Preventive health care						
Expenditures US $ (x 1 million)	899	7,410	850	420	893	333
Expenditures ECU (x 1 million)	757	6,253	716	355	753	281

Table 19.1 (end)
Block III health care expenditures 1995 (Summary of the Bilateral Comparison)

	Netherlands	Denmark	Netherlands	France	Netherlands	Switzerland	Netherlands	Belgium
	1995		1995		1995		1995	
BCP expenditures on Block III: Preventive health care								
Expenditures US $ (x 1 million)	1,137	522	1,137	3,238	1,044	539	1,131	378
Expenditures ECU (x 1 million)	872	399	872	2,474	800	410	867	289

19.3 *Additions & Deductions*

Taking the same procedures and methods into account as presented in the composition of the CCP on Block II, the following remarks can be made in the field of preventive health.

Provisions or activities added to the BCP on prevention are limited to the activities in the field of the Fight against smoking.

The provisions on Drinking water surveillance and Environmental hygiene are deducted from the BCP on prevention.

Environmental hygiene is taken out of the CCP because in Germany, France and Switzerland these activities are not counted as health care activities. In Denmark one amount has been supplied for Environmental hygiene and Drinking water surveillance, so only for the Netherlands separate data in the Health Accounts are available.

The reasons for taking out Drinking water surveillance are that in some countries (France and Switzerland) Drinking water surveillance is no part of the health accounts and no data are supplied for this subject. In Denmark it is combined with Environmental hygiene.

19.4 *Towards a CCP on Block III: Prevention*

Table 19.2
Towards a CCP on Block III health care, 1994 (US $)

	Netherlands	Germany	Netherlands	Switzerland	Netherlands	Belgium
	1994		1994		1994	
	US $ (x 1 million)					
BCP Block III	899	7,410	850	420	893	333
Additions					5	17
Deductions	49	485			49	24
CCP Block III	850	6,926	850	420	850	327

Table 19.2 (end)
Towards a CCP on Block III health care, 1995 (US $)

	Nether-lands	Den-mark	Nether-lands	France	Nether-lands	Switzer-land	Nether-lands	Belgium
	1995		1995		1995		1995	
	US $ (x 1 million)							
BCP Block III	1,137	522	1,137	3,238	1,044	539	1,131	378
Additions							6	20
Deductions	93	23	93	40			93	18
CCP Block III	1,044	499	1,044	3,198	1,044	539	1,044	380

Not only is the number of provisions or activities deducted and added is very small, the amounts of expenditures involved are even smaller. The additions amount to $ 6 million for the Netherlands and $ 20 million for Belgium (1995).
A substantial amount is deducted only for Germany, $ 485 million. For all other countries the deductions are less than 100 million US $ in 1995 and even less than $ 50 million in 1994.

19.5 *The results of the CCP on preventive health care*

In this paragraph the results of the CCP for the six countries involved are described.

Table 19.3
BCP and CCP on Block III health care, 1994, 1995 (% of GDP)

	Year	BCP Block III	Difference [1]	CCP Block III	Difference [1]
The Netherlands	1995	0.29		0.26	
Denmark		0.30	0.01	0.29	0.03
The Netherlands	1994	0.27		0.25	
Germany		0.36	0.09	0.34	0.09
The Netherlands	1995	0.29		0.26	
France		0.21	–0.08	0.21	–0.05
The Netherlands	1994	0.25		0.25	
Switzerland		0.16	–0.09	0.16	–0.09
The Netherlands	1995	0.26		0.26	
Switzerland		0.18	–0.08	0.18	–0.08
The Netherlands	1994	0.27		0.25	
Belgium		0.15	–0.12	0.14	–0.11
The Netherlands	1995	0.31		0.26	
Belgium		0.14	–0.15	0.14	–0.12

[1] Difference in percentagepoints with respect to the Netherlands.

The share of prevention measured in percentages of GDP is very small, because the amounts devoted to prevention as a separate activity or provision are very small in the participating countries.

The differences between the various BCP's are small; the differences between the countries in the CCP are small as well. By and large every participant spent about 0.3 percent of its GDP on separately presented preventive activities. Belgium and Switzerland are the two countries reporting the least spending on prevention as a separate activity (with 0.14 and 0.16 percent of GDP respectively in 1994).

In the table below the results measured in US $ per capita and ECU per capita are presented.

Table 19.4
CCP on Block III: Preventive health care, 1994, 1995 (US $ & ECU per capita)

	Year	Expenditures per capita	
		US $	Ecu
The Netherlands	1995	67	52
Denmark		96	73
The Netherlands	1994	55	47
Germany		85	72
The Netherlands	1995	67	52
France		55	42
The Netherlands	1994	55	47
Switzerland		60	50
The Netherlands	1995	67	52
Switzerland		75	57
The Netherlands	1994	55	47
Belgium		32	27
The Netherlands	1995	67	52
Belgium		38	29

The expenditures on prevention vary between US $ 32 and US $ 96 per capita. The lowest amount per capita is spent in Belgium 1994; the highest amount in Denmark 1995.

In the final part of this paragraph the added results of the constructed CCP's on Block II and Block III will be compared to the data as supplied on the OECD Health data bank 1997.

Table 19.5
OECD Ambulatory care and CCP on Block II & Block III compared, 1994, 1995 (% of GDP)

	Year	OECD Ambulatory care		CCP Block II & Block III	
			Difference [1]		Difference [1]
The Netherlands	1995	2.47		1.62	
Denmark		1.20	–1.27	1.5	–0.15
The Netherlands	1994	2.51		1.65	
Germany		3.06	0.55	3.30	1.65
The Netherlands	1995	2.47		1.62	
France		2.63	0.16	2.61	0.99
The Netherlands	1994	2.51		1.65	
Switzerland		3.60	1.09	2.78	1.13
The Netherlands	1995	2.47		1.62	
Switzerland		3.67	1.20	2.67	1.05
The Netherlands	1994	2.51		1.65	
Belgium		2.97	0.46	1.61	–0.04
The Netherlands	1995	2.47		1.62	
Belgium		3.02	0.55	1.65	0.03

[1] Difference in percentagepoints with respect to the Netherlands.

The OECD Health data bank shows that all countries spent between 2.5 and 3.0 percent of their GDP on ambulatory care. The exception being Denmark with a low of 1.2 percent of GDP and Switzerland with a high of 3.6 percent of GDP.

Looking at the data of the results of the combined Blocks II and III the spending of the countries on Block II and Block III combined is within a small range. The lowest recorded percentage is 1.50 percent of GDP in Denmark in1995 and the highest is 3.30 percent of GDP in Germany in 1995.

The high percentage on Block II and Block III combined for Germany is what can be expected because Germany is known for its more importance the ambulatory care sector. In Denmark this sector is of relative less importance than in the other countries. The rather low score of the Netherlands is caused by the transfer of a large share of the expenditures of Specialists practices from Block II: Extramural health to Block I: Intramural health care. If this transfer had not been carried out the share of Block II and Block III combined for the Netherlands would have been around 2.5% of GDP as well.

The results of the OECD on Ambulatory care expressed in shares of GDP and the combined results of Blocks II and III will be presented in graph 19.1.

Graph 19.1 Block II & Block III health care: OECD and CCP compared, 1994, 1995 (% of GDP)

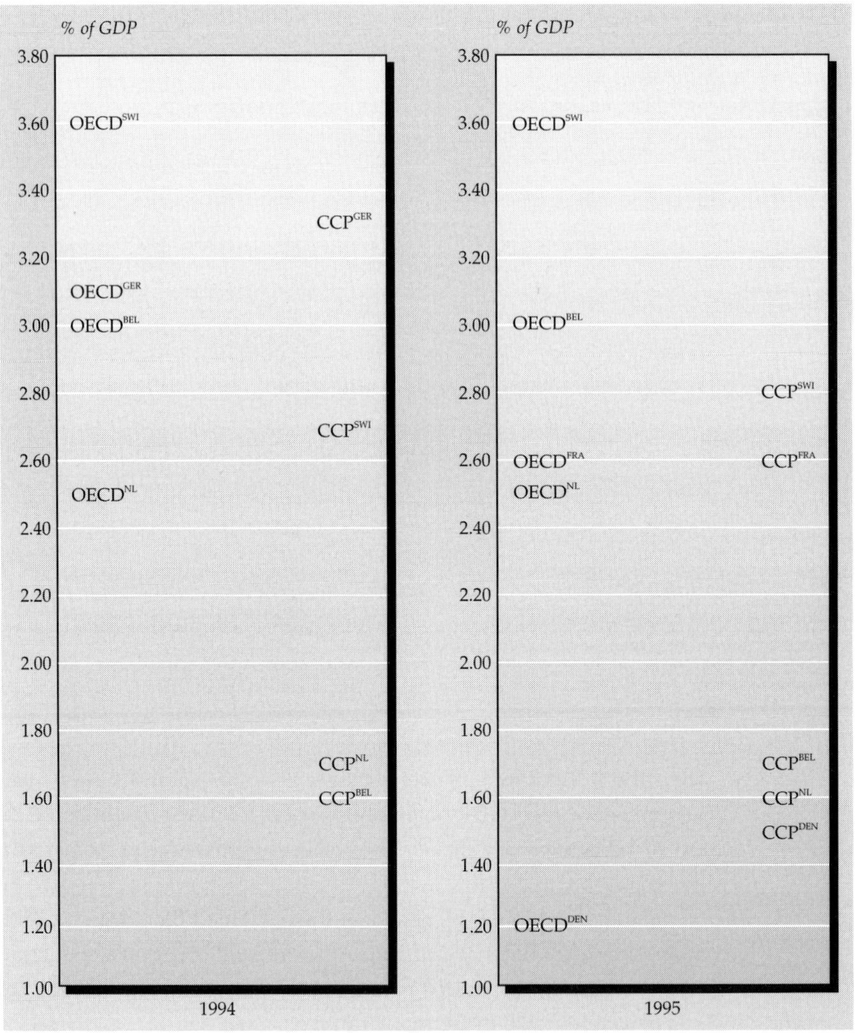

Looking at graph 19.1 it is not surprising that the data in the CCP on the combined Blocks II and III are closer together than the data in the OECD Health data bank. The Netherlands however is an exception due to the fact that about 84 percent of the expenditures of Specialists is transferred to Block I (in the OECD data the expenditures of all independent specialists are included in ambulatory care).

20. Common Comparable Package Block IV: Medical goods

20.1 *Introduction*

In this short chapter the bilateral packages on Block IV: medical goods are "processed" to reach a CCP on Block IV: medical goods.

In the whole area the one real problem is the amount of expenditures on Therapeutic appliances of Switzerland. Because these expenditures are included in the Other ambulatory health care services (without SPITEX) two options are open, i.e. calculating an amount for Therapeutic appliances and excluding that amount from Block II: Extramural health care or leaving the Other ambulatory health care services (without SPITEX) as it is and Therapeutic appliances as well.

We chose this first option and made a calculation for the Therapeutic appliances. The amount is transferred from Block II: Extramural health care to Block IV: Medical goods in order to get more comparability both for the package in Block IV and in Block II.

20.2 *Towards a CCP on Block IV: Medical goods*

The results of the Bilateral Packages are presented in the table below, followed by the Common Comparable Package on Medical goods.

Table 20.1
Towards a CCP on Block IV health care, 1994 (US $)

	Netherlands	Germany	Netherlands	Switzerland	Netherlands	Belgium
	1994		1994		1994	
	US $ (x 1 million)					
BCP Block IV	3,991	35,246	3,991	2,751	3,991	3,642
Additions						
Deductions						
CCP Block IV	3,991	35,246	3,991	2,751	3,991	3,642

Table 20.1 (end)
Towards a CCP on Block IV health care, 1995 (US $)

	Netherlands	Denmark	Netherlands	France	Netherlands	Switzerland	Netherlands	Belgium
	1995		1995		1995		1995	
	US $ (x 1 million)							
BCP Block IV	4,854	1,553	4,854	29,413	4,854	3,410	4,854	4,371
Additions								
Deductions								
CCP Block IV	4,854	1,553	4,854	29,413	4,854	3,410	4,854	4,371

Based on the material at hand, ranging from country profiles, lists of activities and the annotated lists of expenditures on provisions, it cannot be determined if there should be any additions or deductions.

Because no additions or deductions were necessary, the BCP on Medical goods equals the CCP on Medical goods.

21. Construction of the Common Comparable Package of health care

21.1 Introduction

In this final chapter on the construction of the Common Comparable Packages an attempt is made to present the total CCP of health care in the participating countries. The total CCP consists of the CCP on Block I: Intramural health care, the CCP on Block II: Extramural, the CCP on Block III: Preventive health care and the CCP on Block IV: Medical goods. From Block·V: Other services only the section on Administration is added to create a total on health care, very much in line with the contents of health care in de the participating countries.

Although the links between the activities and provisions in Block II and Block III are very strong, and it is in some cases impossible to separate them, it was strongly advised to create two different CCP Blocks.

The problem of the Therapeutic appliances for Switzerland is solved in the CCP on Medical goods. Therapeutic appliances for Switzerland are calculated and taken out of the CCP on Block II health care and transferred to Block IV.
On the subject of Other services the problems with lacking data have to be solved, especially in the field of the expenditures on Research & Development. To a lesser extent the same problem exists in the area of Education & Training. So just the Administration expenditures remain of the Other services to be included in the CCP approach.

21.2 The CCP of health care

The first preliminary constructed CCP results are presented in the table below.

Table 21.1
Expenditures on the total CCP of health care, 1994 (US $)

	Netherlands	Germany	Switzerland	Belgium
	1994	1994	1994	1994
CCP Block I	15,688	92,286	12,126	8,617
CCP Block II	4,718	60,749	6,543	3,884
CCP Block III	850	6,926	420	327
CCP Block IV	3,991	35,246	2,751	3,642
CCP "Administration"	1,277	4,420	1,464	658
CCP Health care	26,523	206,713	23,303	16,627

Table 21.1 (end)
Expenditures on the total CCP of health care, 1995 (US $)

	Netherlands	Denmark	France	Switzerland	Belgium
	1995	1995	1995	1995	1995
CCP Block I	18,454	8,209	81,241	14,446	10,318
CCP Block II	5,373	2,097	36,916	7,976	4,119
CCP Block III	1,044	499	3,198	539	380
CCP Block IV	4,954	1,533	29,413	3,410	4,371
CCP "Administration"	1,489	124	9,245	1,880	740
CCP Health care	31,214	12,481	160,012	28,251	19,928

The data as supplied in the table above has a limited meaning in a comparable way. For that reason in the graphs below (graph 21.1 and graph 21.2) the data on the CCP Blocks are presented as shares in the total of health care.

Graph 21.1 Percentage shares of Block I to Block IV & Administration in total CCP, 1994

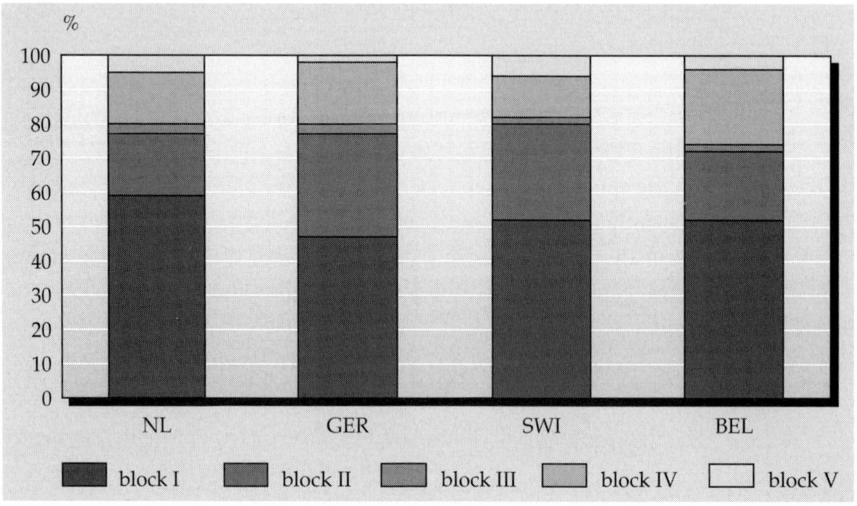

In all countries Block I is of great importance in the total of health care (between 50 and 60 percent). In Denmark Block I represents 66 percent of the total CCP, in Germany on the contrary Block I only represents 46 percent. Block II is of great importance in Germany (30 percent) followed by Switzerland (28 percent). In all other countries it is about 17 percent of the total of CCP. Block III – in all countries politically very important – only takes between 2 and 4 percent of total CCP expenditures. Block IV on medical goods ranges between 12 (Switzerland) and 19 percent (Belgium) of total CCP.

Graph 21.2 **Percentage shares of Block I to Block IV & Administration in total CCP, 1995**

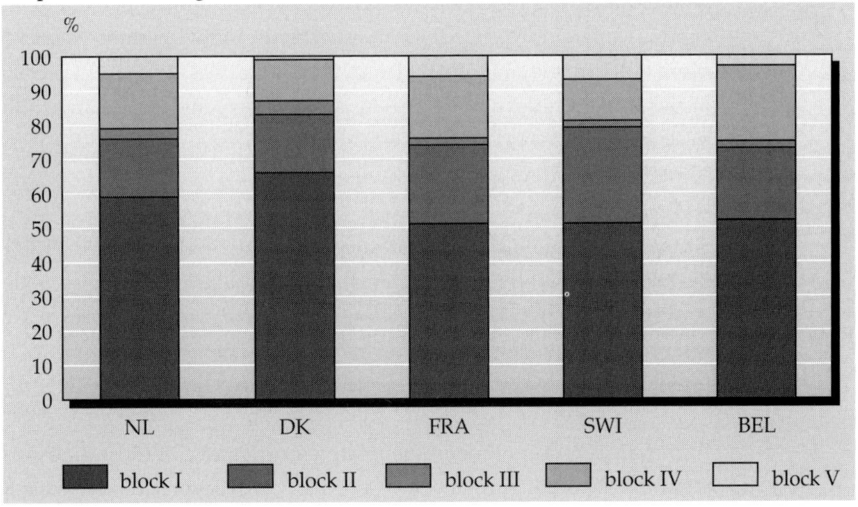

In the table below the expenditures on the total CCP are expressed in US dollars and in ECU per capita.

Table 21.2
CCP on total health care, 1994 (US $ & ECU per capita)

	Year	Expenditures per capita	
		US $	Ecu
The Netherlands	1995	2,016	1,546
Denmark		2,350	1,825
The Netherlands	1994	1,724	1,453
Germany		2,539	2,507
The Netherlands	1995	2,016	1,546
France		2,754	2,104
The Netherlands	1994	1,724	1,453
Switzerland		3,312	2,800
The Netherlands	1995	2,016	1,546
Switzerland		3,942	3,001
The Netherlands	1994	1,724	1,453
Belgium		1,664	1,387
The Netherlands	1995	2,016	1,546
Belgium		1,968	1,504

Comparing the amounts spent on health (CCP) in the participating countries the differences do not seem big. In the Netherlands around $ 2,000 per capita is included in the CCP on Health ($ 1,724 in 1994 and $ 2,016 in 1995), in Germany and France $ 2,539 respectively $ 2,754. The differences in percentages with respect to the

Netherlands for France and in Germany reveal that 37 percent and 47 percent per capita is spent more, than in the Netherlands. In Switzerland a considerable amount more is spent on the CCP on Health $ 3,304 in 1994 (94 percent per capita more than in the Netherlands) and $ 3,886 in 1995 (93 percent more than in the Netherlands). In Belgium $ 1,644 per capita is spent on health in 1994 and $ 1,968 in 1995 (about 70 percent less than in the Netherlands).

A comparison of two years is possible for the Netherlands, Switzerland and Belgium. Because the ECU is less volatile than the dollar, the ECU is better suited for a comparison of two years. In the Netherlands the expenditures per capita grew by 6.3 percent from 1994 to 1995. In Switzerland the growth was only 5.9 percent and in Belgium it was 8.5 percent considerably more than in the Netherlands.

A graphic representation of the relative importance of the various Blocks per capita is provided in the graphs below, one for 1994 (graph 21.3) and one for 1995 (graph 21.4).

Graph 21.3 Expenditures per capita of Block I to Block IV & Administration, 1994

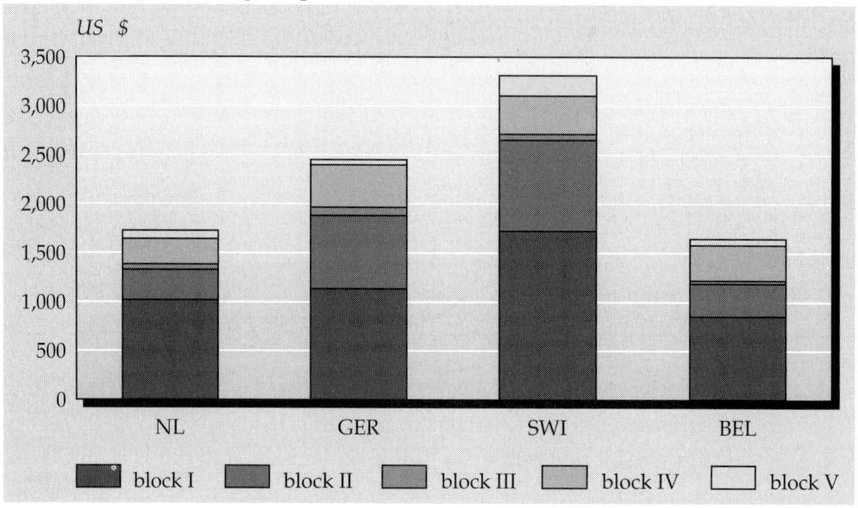

Graph 21.4 Expenditures per capita of Block I to Block IV & Administration, 1995

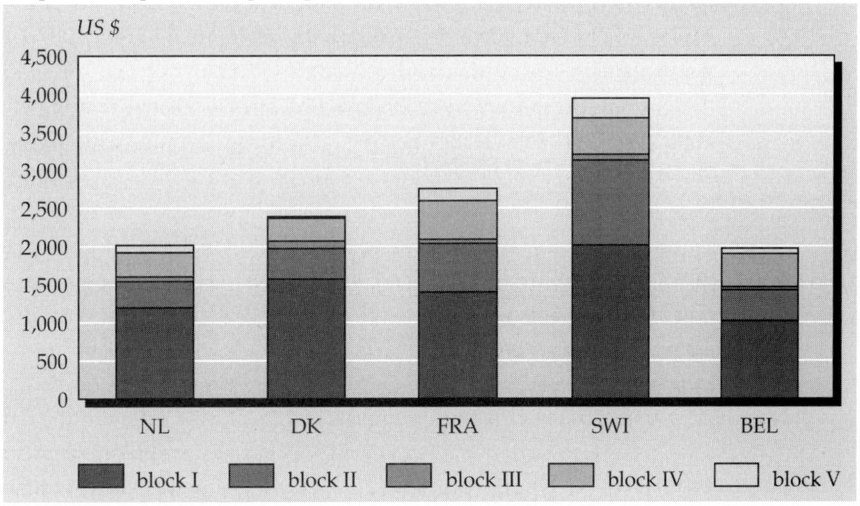

In table 21.3 the expenditures (shares of GDP) originating from the OECD and the CCP-project are compared.

Table 21.3
Total health care expenditures: OECD and total CCP compared, 1994, 1995 (% of GDP)

	Year	OECD Total Health care		CCP Total	
			Difference [1]		Difference [1]
The Netherlands	1995	8.8		7.9	
Denmark		6.4	–2.4	7.2	–0.7
The Netherlands	1994	8.8		7.9	
Germany		10.3	1.5	9.7	1.8
The Netherlands	1995	8.8		7.9	
France		9.9	1.1	10.4	2.5
The Netherlands	1994	8.8		7.9	
Switzerland		9.6	0.8	9.1	1.2
The Netherlands	1995	8.8		7.9	
Switzerland		9.8	1.0	9.2	1.3
The Netherlands	1994	8.8		7.9	
Belgium		8.1	–0.7	7.3	–0.6
The Netherlands	1995	8.8		7.9	
Belgium		8.0	–0.8	7.4	–0.5

[1] Difference in percentagepoints with respect to the Netherlands.

Expressed in percentages of GDP the Netherlands spent 7.9 percent on the CCP on Health. In Germany 1.8 percentage points more, in France 3.0 percentage points more than in the Netherlands. Switzerland compared to the Netherlands spent 1.1 percentage point more in 1994 and 1.2 in 1995. Denmark and Belgium spent less than the Netherlands (0.5 and 0.7 percentage points respectively in 1995). The difference between France and the other participants can to a certain extent be explained by the treatment of the nursing home care and the administration. The calculation of the Nursing home care and the additionally supplied data on the Administration in France lead to an addition of 0.6 percent of GDP in the expenditures. This results in 10.4 percent of GDP devoted tot health care in the CCP of France.

This becomes clear in comparing the results of the CCP with the data presented in the OECD Health data bank. In the OECD health data bank France spent 9.9 percent of its GDP on Health compared to 8.8 percent for the Netherlands. The difference between France and the Netherlands is 1.1 percentage point, but this is much less than the difference in the CCP on health between the two countries (2.5 percentage points).

For five participants (the Netherlands, Germany, Denmark, Switzerland and Belgium) the share devoted to health is smaller in the CCP approach than in the data supplied in the OECD health data bank. For the other two countries (Denmark and France) the results in the CCP-approach are higher than the results in the OECD health data bank.

For Belgium the difference between OECD data and the CCP is 0.8 in 1994 and 0.6 percentage points in 1995; for Switzerland 0.6 percentage points in 1994 and 0.7 in 1995. For Germany the difference is 0.7 percentage point the same as for Denmark. For the Netherlands the difference is 0.8 percentage points. For France the difference between the OECD and the CCP is 1 percentage point.

Comparing the results in the CCP approach (as percentages of GDP) the packages are more uniform, ranging from 7.1% for Denmark to 10.9 % for the France. Leaving out the highest and the lowest (France and Denmark), the range is limited from 7.4 percent (Belgium) to 9.6 percent in Germany.

Finally in the last graph (graph 21.5) the relative positions of the OECD data and the CCP data are presented for the participating countries.

Graph 21.5 Expenditures on health care: OECD, BCP and CCP compared, 1994, 1995 (% of GDP)

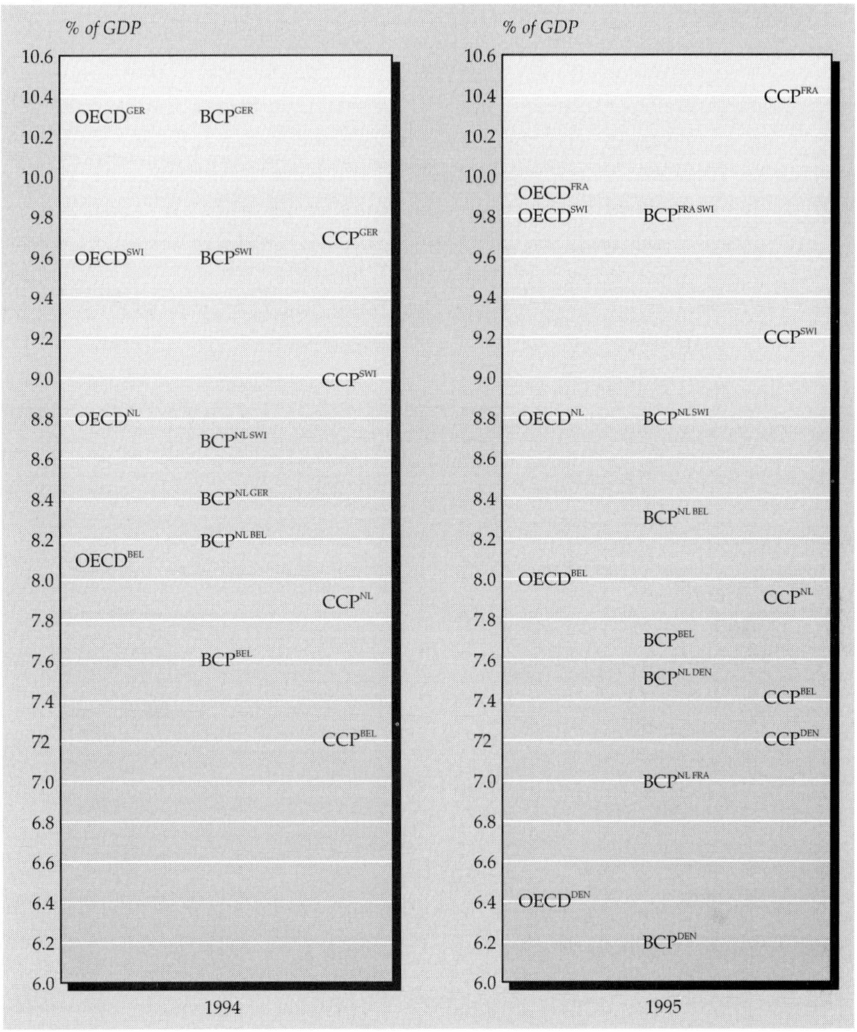

22. Evaluation

22.1 Introduction

At the end of the project "international comparison of health care data", the main results are reviewed briefly. The starting point for the evaluation of this phase of the project is the aims and objectives as mentioned in section 1 of chapter 2. First however the results of the comparisons of Phase II are evaluated briefly.

22.2 Results of Phase 2 based on the data available

In these paragraphs the results of the various chapters are presented, starting with chapter 9 the "general framework", followed by the Bilateral Comparisons (Chapters 10 to 14) and ending with the Common Comparable Packages (chapters 16 to 21).

- Conclusions based on the General framework (chapter 9).

Comparing the Gross Domestic Product (GDP) per capita of all six participating countries, the Netherlands showed the lowest GDP per capita of all (US $ 21,896 in 1994 and US $ 25,476 in 1995). Switzerland on the other hand performed best with a GDP per capita of US $ 36,607 in 1994 and US $ 42,811 in 1995.

Comparing the data on GDP expressed in US dollars and in Purchasing Power Parities (PPP) it was clear that only for Switzerland and Denmark it was relevant in which value the data are expressed. In Denmark the difference in GDP per capita expressed in US dollars and PPP was 54 percent; in Switzerland this difference was 53 percent in 1994 and 75 percent in 1995. The difference between these two measures was much smaller in the other countries. The difference ranged between 12 percent in Belgium, 17 percent for the Netherlands 28 percent for Germany in 1994, to 28 percent for Denmark, 29 percent for the Netherlands, 33 percent for France in 1995.

However large these difference are in one country, in Bilateral Comparisons the relative difference between two countries is relevant. Taking this into account only for Denmark and Switzerland it was relevant in which measure the data are expressed.

Denmark devoted 6.4 percent of GDP to health care and Germany 10.3 percent according to the OECD Health data bank, a difference in spending of 3.9 percentage points for two highly developed countries in Western Europe. Expressed in US dollars per capita the differences were large as well, ranging in 1994 from $ 1,858 in Belgium to $ 3,578 in Switzerland, almost twice as much (92 percent exactly). Serious doubts on the comparability of the contents of these packages are valid.

- Bilateral Comparisons (chapters 10 to 14).

The results in chapter 10, the BCP on Block I: Intramural health care, showed that Belgium was the only country to spend less per capita than the Netherlands. In Belgium 18 percent (1994) less was spent on Block I. In all other countries more was spent on Block I. In Germany 9 percent, in Denmark 13 percent and in France 26 percent. Switzerland however spent 69 percent more per capita both in 1994 and 1995 than the Netherlands.

Because provisions on Block II: Extramural health care and Block III: prevention were very difficult to separate in money terms and the influence of Block III on the total of Block II and Block III was small, these two Blocks were presented together.

Belgium spent about the same amount per capita on Block II and Block III combined as the Netherlands (1 percent more in 1994 and 5 percent more in 1995). For all other countries the differences were much larger. France spent 68 percent more per capita. Germany spent almost double the amount per capita (92 percent more) of the Netherlands. In Switzerland however 131 percent more per capita was spent than in the Netherlands in 1994.

In chapter 13 the BCP on Medical goods, Block IV, was described. In the area of medical goods Denmark spent 7 percent less than the Netherlands. All other participants spent more per capita, ranging from 39 percent in Belgium (1994) to 61 percent in France (1995).

In chapter 14 the attempted comparisons on Block V: Other services were presented. Other services comprise the expenditures on Research & Development, Education & Training and Administration. Although the expenditures on R&D should in theory be comparable for some countries (the Netherlands–Germany to a certain extent, and the Netherlands–France) it was shown in that chapter that comparability is not present in the data. The same result was imminent on the comparison of the expenditures on Education & Training (comparable in theory, but not comparable in actual data). So from chapter 14 on Other services only the Administration was included in the comparison.

In chapter 15 the Input supplied by the participants on the subject of health care and health care related activities were compared to the results of the Bilateral Comparisons. Only in the Bilateral Comparison of the Netherlands and Switzerland 100 percent was used for both countries. Belgium was the only country for which more than 100 per cent of the Input was used in the Bilateral Comparison, caused by the Additional payments (included in the BCP but not a part on the Input file concerning health care). in the other three comparisons less than 100 percent of the

Input was used, ranging from 79 percent in the case of France and 95 percent in the case of Germany.

- Common Comparable Packages (chapters 17 to 20).

In chapter 17 to 20 the Common Comparable Packages were presented on the various Blocks (Block I to Block IV), followed by a chapter on the construction of a CCP on the total health care (chapter 21). In the construction of a CCP Additions and Deductions were necessary. In the summary on the results first these Additions and Deductions will be presented, followed by the results of the CCP's of the various Blocks.

Additions

In Block I the additions ranged from $ 404 million in Belgium in 1994 (4.9 percent of the BCP) to $ 15,313 million in France in 1995 (23 percent of the BCP). No additions were needed in the construction of the CCP of Block I: Intramural health care for the BCP of the Netherlands and Germany (1994).

The additions in Block II: Extramural health care ranged from $ 8 million in Belgium in 1994 (0.2 percent of the BCP) to $ 244 million for the Netherlands (3.4 percent) in the BCP with Switzerland in 1995. No additions in Block II were necessary in France, Denmark (both 1995) and Germany (1994).

In Block III on Prevention additions were limited to $ 5 million (0.6 percent for the Netherlands) in the BCP with Belgium in 1994. For Belgium the additions amounted to $ 17 million (being 5.1 percent of the BCP) in the same year. All other countries needed no additional corrections.

Deductions

In Block I the deductions ranged from $ 29 million for the Netherlands (0.2 percent) in the BCP with Belgium in 1994 to $ 2,200 million for the Netherlands (11 percent) in the BCP with Switzerland in 1995. No deductions in Block I were necessary for Denmark (1995), Germany (1994) and Belgium (1994 and 1995).

In Block II for every country deductions were needed. The deductions ranged from $ 552 million for the Netherlands (9.3 percent) in the BCP with France in 1995 to $ 6,602 million for Germany in 1994 (9.8 percent of the BCP).

Only for Switzerland no deductions in Block III on prevention were necessary. In the other countries the deductions ranged from $ 18 million in Belgium (4.8 percent of the BCP) in 1995 to $ 485 million in Germany (6.5 percent) in 1994.

No additions and deductions were necessary In Block IV on Medical goods, which means that the results presented in the BCP on Block IV were equal to the results of the CCP on Block IV. For Switzerland the amount added to Block IV (partially transferred from Block II) was already introduced in the construction of the BCP for Switzerland.

Results of the Common Comparable Packages

The results of the CCP on Block I: Intramural health care showed that Belgium still spent less per capita than the Netherlands. In 1994 16 percent per capita is spent less in Belgium and 15 percent in 1995. In the BCP the difference was 18 percent for 1994 and 16 percent for 1995. All the other countries spent more. Germany spent 9 percent more (in the BCP the difference was 9 percent as well), Switzerland spent 68 percent per capita more than the Netherlands in both years (in the BCP Switzerland spent 69 percent more). Only for Denmark the difference with the BCP results were more pronounced. In the CCP Denmark spent 30 percent per capita more on Block I compared to the Netherlands; in the BCP Denmark spent only 13 percent more.

In the CCP on Block II and Block III the differences with the Bilateral Comparisons were not big. Belgium spent 1 percent more than the Netherlands on the CCP per capita in 1994 and 7 percent in 1995. In the BCP of these two Blocks combined Belgium spent 1 percent more in 1994 and only 5 percent in 1995 than the Netherlands. Denmark spent 27 percent per capita more on the CCP on Block II and Block III combined in 1995 (the difference in the BCP was 17 percent). Germany spent 127 percent more in the CCP; in the BCP the excess spending compared to the Netherlands was 92 percent. In France the difference with the Netherlands was 67 percent per capita (in the BCP the difference was 68 percent). The largest difference was still recorded in Switzerland. In Switzerland 173 percent was spent more on the CCP in these Blocks (in 1994) than in the Netherlands (in the BCP of 1994 the difference was 131 per capita).

As already mentioned no additions and deductions were necessary in the construction of the CCP on Block IV. So the BCP on this Block equaled the CCP on Block IV. The differences ranged from 7 percent spent less in Denmark to 67 percent spent more per capita in Germany.

Chapter 21 dealt with the construction of the CCP of total health care. As might be expected the differences recorded in the various Blocks of the CCP were still present but less pronounced. So the difference in one block of health care was compensated by a less large difference in another block of health care.

Of course Belgium spent less per capita in the total CCP of health care than the Netherlands (4 percent in 1994 and 2 percent in 1995). In Denmark 18 percent is spent more per capita and finally in Switzerland 95 percent (in 1995) is spent more on health than in the Netherlands.

In all countries the importance of Block I was very large, ranging from 46 percent in Germany (1994) to 66 percent in Denmark (1995). In the Netherlands the importance of Block I was 59 percent in the total CCP; in Belgium and Switzerland 52 percent in 1994. In Germany Block II and Block III combined were responsible for 35 percent of the expenditures, in Switzerland for 30 percent and in France 25 percent. In Belgium and the Netherlands these two Blocks were responsible for 23 percent and 20 percent respectively in 1995. Medical goods (Block IV) were accountable for 12 percent in Switzerland (1994), 18 percent in Germany (1994) and France (1995) and 22 percent in Belgium (in both years). In the Netherlands Block IV was responsible for 15 percent (1994) and 16 percent (1995). Administration expenditures, the last item in the CCP, was responsible for a share of 4 percent in Belgium (1994 and 1995), 5 percent in the Netherlands (1994) and 6 percent in Switzerland (1994) and in France (1995). In Germany Administration was accountable for 2 percent of the total expenditures of the CCP which is low, but in Denmark Administration was only 1 percent, very low compared to the highest share recorded in Switzerland and France (6 percent).

Generalised conclusions of Phase II

- Contrary to the construction of the Bilateral Comparable Packages in Phase I, calculations were necessary in this Phase on extramural health care, prevention and medical goods even in the construction of the Bilateral Comparable Packages. To a large extent this is caused by the complexity of the field and the large heterogeneity of activities and providers.
- The approach of the CCP method supplies more uniform, comparable results, even in such heterogeneous sectors as extramural health care, prevention and medical goods.
- The large importance of intramural health care is not always accompanied by an opposite or minor importance of the non-intramural health care sectors. Only in Germany a relative small intramural sector is compensated by a large non-intramural sector. In France however a large intramural sector is accompanied by a large non-intramural sector.

22.3 *Evaluation of aims and objectives*

- Determination of the boundaries of health care.

In determining the boundaries of health care the country profiles (chapter 3 to chapter 8) were used extensively. The country profiles supplied an overview of the health care system in all its aspects of a country. More detailed information was acquired through the matrices in which participants indicated whether care provisions existed or not and belonged to the health care systems or not. The results provide a clear overview of the boundaries of health care of the participating countries (see Annex 2.3).

- Development of the methodology and model for international comparison.

The most important feature of the development of the methodology is the notion that activities are the basic starting point. Based on these activities it was possible to describe provisions and the production factors (expenditures) connected with them. The bilateral comparisons were carried out at the level of health care provisions. Principally this method can be used successfully in all sectors of health care and for non-financial variables as well.

- Comparison of the health care systems of the participating countries by means of a reference model.

A Common Comparable Package (CCP) was constructed based on the bilateral comparisons. The CCP consists of provisions selected from the lists of provisions used in the bilateral comparisons. Those selected provisions are counted as part of the common health care systems of the participating countries.
Our conclusion is that the CCP-approach can be used as a reference: a common concept to be used in international comparisons.

22.4 *Some final remarks:*

- The intention of the pragmatic approach by Statistics Netherlands was to leave intact definitions at national level and not to impose uniform definitions, as is common practice in international data collection. The possibilities for comparison have been enlarged by annotations and comments facilitating better understanding of the data.
- The project offered the opportunity to benefit from the value of interaction especially within the network of experts and to establish increasing consensus and, as a consequence, a better understanding of the meaning of data. However, not all problems were solved. R&D and E&T e.g. were too difficult to be compared. In the field of the transport of patients the availability and quality of data made comparison difficult (see the report on "Transport of patients").
- The participating countries are encouraged to compare their own data with other countries, using the same methods; by discussing the results together, so that the influence of the so-called ethnocentric judgements might be eliminated and more experience in improving the methods will be acquired.
- Not only among participating countries interest was raised in the topic of international comparison of health care data and the methods applied. Also other countries as well as international organisations have taken further steps in this

field. This justifies the expectation, that although this project – financed by the Dutch Ministry of Health, Welfare and Sports – came to an end, the process of improving international comparison of health care data will be continued more or less along the same lines.

Annexes

Annex 2.1: Participants Network of Experts

Annex 2.1.1: Participants Network of Experts Phase I, 1994–1995

Dr. J. Branckaerts †
Ministerie van Volksgezondheid
en Leefmilieu
Brussel, Belgium

Dr. G. Brückner
Statistisches Bundesamt, VII D
Wiesbaden, Germany

Mr. R.W. Haneveld
Ministerie van VWS
Rijswijk, The Netherlands

Mr. P.E. Hansen
Sundhedsministeriet
København, Denmark

Mr. M.W. Knüppel
EUROSTAT
Luxemburg

Dr. D. v.d. Meer (chairman)
National Hospital Federation
Utrecht, The Netherlands

Mr. A. Nanda
WHO Regional Office for Europe
København, Denmark

Prof. Dr. Jozef Pacolet
Hoger Instituut voor de Arbeid
Leuven, Belgium

Mr. Patrick Pauriche
SESI, Ministère des Affaires Sociales
de la Santé et de la Ville
Paris, France

Mr. J.P. Poullier
OECD
Paris, France

Dr. Simone Sandier
CREDES
Paris, France

Dr. Markus Schneider
BASYS
Augsburg, Germany

Mr. Jes Søgaard
Centre for Health and Social Policy
Odense, Denmark

Dr. Marc Wyss
Bundesamt für Statistik
Bern, Switzerland

Annex 2.1.2: Participants Network of Experts Phase II, 1996–1997

Mr. J.T.P. Bonte
(chairman)
EUROSTAT
Luxembourg, Luxemburg

Dr. G. Brückner
Statistisches Bundesamt, VII D
Wiesbaden, Germany

Mr. H. Haveman
(until Jan 1st 1997)
Mr. R.A.G. van Puijenbroek
(from Jan 1st 1997)
Ministerie van Volksgezondheid, Welzijn en Sport
Rijswijk, The Netherlands

Mr. P.E. Hansen
Mrs. M Kruse
Sundhedsministeriet
København, Denmark

Dr. M Huber
OECD
Paris, France

Mr. T. Montserrat
EUROSTAT
Luxembourg, Luxemburg

Mr. A. Nanda
WHO Regional Office for Europe
Copenhagen, Denmark

Dr. H. Van Oyen
Instituut voor Hygiëne en Epidemiologie
Brussel, Belgium

Prof. Dr. Jozef Pacolet
Hoger Instituut voor de Arbeid
Leuven, Belgium

Mr. Patrick Pauriche
SESI, Ministère du Travail et des Affaires Sociales
Paris, France

Mrs V. Paris
CREDES
Paris, France

Dr. Markus Schneider
BASYS
Augsburg, Germany

Mr. R. Wagener
Inspection Générale de la Sécurité sociale
Luxembourg, Luxembourg

Dr. Marc Wyss
(until October 1st 1997)
Dr. T. Spuhler
(from October 1st 1997)
Bundesamt für Statistik
Bern, Switzerland

Annex 2.2: List of activities in health care services

Activities (tied to patients):

General medical treatment

General dentistry

Specialised medical treatment:

- internal medicine
- surgery
- obstetrics & gynaecology
- otorhinolaryngology
- ophthalmology
- paediatrics
- dermatology
- allergology
- anaesthesiology
- cardiology
- cardiopulmonal surgery
- gastro-enterology
- clinical chemistry
- clinical geriatrics
- diseases of lung and tuberculosis
- medical microbiology
- neurosurgery
- neurology
- nuclear medicine
- orthopaedics
- pathology
- plastic surgery
- psychiatry
- radiodiagnostics
- radiotherapy
- rheumatology
- rehabilitation
- urology

Other specialisms:

- clinical genetics
- mouth diseases and jawsurgery
- orthodontics
- clinical physiology
- clinical physic
- clinical psycholog

Specialisms supplemented by participants:
- endocrinology
- chemotherapy
- angiology
- nephrology
- forensic medicine
- neonatology
- psychogeriatrics
- anthroposofic treatment
- labour safety
- preventive medicine
- clinical pharmacology
- oncology
- haematology

Nursing:
- qualified home nursing
- home care

Mother and child care:
- care of midwives
- maternity home care

Other activities (directly tied to patients):
- emergency care/first aid
- function tests
- laboratory tests
- supply of pharmaceuticals
- supply of therapeutic appliances
- speech therapy
- dietetic advice
- dental hygiene
- podotherapy
- medical welfare
- pastoral care
- transport of patients

Physical training:
- physiotherapy
- ergonomic therapy
- movement therapy

Mental treatment and training:
- psychotherapy
- psychosocial diagnostics
- psychosocial treatment
- pedagogic diagnostics
- pedagogic training
- orthodidactic diagnostics

Other activities (not directly tied to patients):
- training of personnel
- accomodation of personnel
- maintenance of buildings, terrain's & installations
- catering
- administration
- medical registration
- support of family care
- support of home care

Features of care:
- topclinical care
- clinical care
- day and/or night treatment
- hospital outpatient department
- consultation room visits
- home visits
- consultation by telephone
- home care

Forms of lodging:
- residential care
- durable accomodation
- short term admission
- day nursing
- night care
- holiday relief

Preventive health care activities:

health protection:
- nutritional surveillance
- drinking water surveillance
- environmental hygiene/surveillance

health promotion:

- health education and information
- fight against smoking
- fight against alcohol and drugs abuse
- prevention of accidents:
  - home
  - leisure
  - traffic
  - work

general prevention of diseases:

- immunisation
- other prevention of infectious diseases
- screening & early detection
  - genetic counselling
  - antenatal assessment/pregnancy control
  - early detection of developmental disorders
  - mass screening on specific diseases (e.g. cervix carcinoma, mamma carcinoma)
  - mass screening on risk factors (e.g. hypertension, cholesterol)
  - periodical, systematic examinations:
    - school health
    - school dental health
    - occupational health

Other services

- training & education of health personnel
  - in universities (medical staff)
  - in schools (medical & paramedical staff)
- research & development in health (pharmaceutical & biomedical)
  - in business enterprises
  - in univerisities
  - in special research centres
- health care administration
  - by local authorities (municipalities, provinces, etc.)
  - central government (departments of health)
  - health insurance boards
  - health insurance funds
  - health insurance bodies
  - private insurance companies

Annex 2.3: Boundaries of health care

An overview of health care provisions in six countries

Provisions indicated as counted in health accounts:	+
Provisions indicated as not counted in health accounts:	–
Provisions indicated as partially counted in health accounts:	p
Provisions indicated as non-existing:	o

Intramural health care services	B	DK	F	G	NL	CH
acute hospital	+	–	+	–	–	+
general hospital	–	+	–	+	+	–
university/teaching hospital	+	+	+	+	+	+
specialized hospital (Fachkrankenhaus)	+	+	+	+	+	+
maternity clinic	+	+	+	+	+	+
anti poison centre	o	o	+	o	o	o
day care services						
hospital day care	+	+	+	+	+	+
oncological and radiotherapeutical day treatment	+	+	+	+	+	+
nurseries for toddlers under medical supervision	o	o	+	o	+	+
abortion clinics	o	o	o	+	–	+
private clinics (daycare only)	o	+	+	–	–	+
day centres for physically disabled	–	–	p	–	+	+
reconvalescence day centres	o	–	p	+	+	+
day centres for the mentally ill	p	p	p	+	+	+
day centres for the mentally deficient	–	–	p	+	+	+
day centres for elderly people	p	–	p	+	p	+
short term recovery homes	+	o	–	+	–	+
long term care institution						
psychiatric hospital	+	+	+	+	+	+
specialized hospital chronically ill (Sonderkrankenhaus)	+	+	+	+	+	+
health spa (Kurort, Cure thermal)	+	+	+	+	o	p
residential care institutions						
institution for the mentally deficient	–	–	p	–	+	p
nursing home	+	–	p	+	+	+
home for the elderly	+	–	p	–	–	+
family replacement homes (youngsters)	–	–	p	–	–	–
home for the sensorily handicapped	–	–	p	–	+	p
medical children's home	o	o	p	o	+	+
other homes	o	–	p	o	+	–

Intramural health care services (continued)	B	DK	F	G	NL	CH
institutions for supervised dwelling						
under medical supervision	+	–	p	o	o	+
under psychotherapeutic supervision	–	–	p	+	p	p
under sociotherapeutic supervision	–	–	p	–	p	+

Extramural health care services	B	DK	F	G	NL	CH
general practitioner	+	+	+	+	+	+
specialist (ambulatory surgery inc.)	+	+	+	+	+	+
dentist	+	+	+	+	+	+
dispensary	+	o	+	o [1)]	o	o
health centre	+	o	+	o [1)]	+	+
hospital out–patient department	+	+	+	+	+	+
physiotherapist/ergonomic therapist	+	+	+	+	+	+
speech therapist	–	–	+	+	+	+
dietician	–	–	–	+	+	+
psychotherapist/psychologist	–	+	–	+	+	+
treatment of alcoholics and drug abusers	+	p	+	+	+	p
medical laboratory	+	+	+	+	+	+
midwife	+	+	+	+	+	+
home/district nurse	+	+	+	+	+	+
home help (family and the elderly)	–	–	–	+ [2)]	+	+
maternity home help	–	+	–	+	+	+
hospital home care	o	o	o	o	+	+
family care of mental patients	–	–	+	+	+	–
alternative medicine (non medical)	–	–	–	+	–	+
anthroposofic medical treatment	–	–	o	+ [3)]	+	–
transport of patients	+	+	+	+	+	p
anti poison centre (for consultation only)	+	o	o	o	+	+

Preventive health care services	B	DK	F	G	NL	CH
Health protection						
nutritional surveillance	+	+	p	p	+	+
drinking water surveillance	+	–	+	p	+	–
environmental hygiene/surveillance	+	–	p	–	–	–
Health promotion						
health education and information	+	p	+	+	+	+
fight against smoking	+	p	+	+	+	+
fight against alcohol and drugs abuse	+	p	+	+	+	+
prevention of accidents:						
home	+	–	+	p	+	+
leisure	+	–	+	p	+	+

Preventive health care services (continued)	B	DK	F	G	NL	CH
traffic	+	–	–	–	–	+
work	+	–	+	+	+	+
General prevention of diseases:						
immunisation	+	+	+	+	+	+
other prevention of infectious diseases	+	+	+	+	+	+
screening & early detection						
genetic counselling	+	+	+	+	+	+
antenatal assessment/pregnancy control	p	+	+	p	+	+
early detection of developmental disorders	p	+	+	+	+	+
mass screening on specific diseases (e.g. cervix carcinoma, mamma carcinoma)	+	+	+	+	+	+
mass screening on risk factors (e.g. hypertension, cholesterol)	–	+	+	+[4)]	+	+
periodical, systematic examinations:						
school health	+	+	+	+	+	+
school dental health	+	+	+	+	+[5)]	+
occupational health	+	–	+	+	+	+

Supply of medical goods

Medical goods by type of product: (division according to data collection in 1992, 1993)	B	DK	F	G	NL	CH
Pharmaceuticals						
prescribed medicines	+	+	+	+	+	+
over the counter medicines	–	+	+	+	p	+
wound dressings etc.	+	+	–	+	p	p
blood and blood products	+	+	+	+	+	+
human products	+	+	+	+	+	+
Therapeutic appliances						
prosthetics/ortheses						
– dental	+	p	+	+	+	+
– maxillofacial	+	p	+	+	+	+
– limb	+	p	+	+	+	+
– other	+	p	+	+	+	+
glasses	+	+	+	+	+	p
other vision aids	+	+	+	+	+	–
hearing aids	+	p	+	+	+	p
orthopedic shoes	+	p	+	+		p
elastic stockings	+	–	–	–	+	–
walking aids	+	p	+	+	+	p

Supply of medical goods (continued)	B	DK	F	G	NL	CH
wigs	+	−	−	p	+	−
personal care materials (e.g.incontinency)	+	−	+	+		p
diabetics aids	+	+	+	+	+	−
medico–technical devices	+	+	+	+	+	+
pacemaker	+	+	+	+	+	+
i.u.d.	+	+	+	+	+	+
Medical goods by supplier: (division according to data collection in 1994, 1995)	B	DK	F	G	NL	CH
Pharmaceuticals supplied by						
Pharmacists	+	p	+	p	+	+
Dispensing general practitioners	+	−	+	+	+	+
Dispensing specialists	+	−	+	+	o	+
Druggists	p	−	−	p	p	p
Therapeutic appliances supplied by						
Dental prothetists	+	p	+	+	+	+
Dental technicians	+	p	+	+	+	+
Prothetist shops	−	p	+	+	+	p
Orthopaedic shoemakers	+	p	p	+	+	p
Orthopaedic shops	+	p	p	+	+	p
Opticians	+	p	+	+	+	p
Hearing aid shops	+	p	p	+	+	p
Other suppliers	p	−	p	+	p	p
Other services	B	DK	F	G	NL	CH
occupational and social rehabilitation	p	−	−	+	−	p
income compensation in case of illness or disability	+	−	p	+	−	−
specific financial support in case of illness or disability	+	−	−	+	−	−
subventions in case of decease	+	−	−	−	o	o
education/training of health care staff						
universities (medical staff)	−	−	+	−	−	−
schools (medical & paramedical professions)	−	+	+	+	−	−
health research (pharmaceutical & biomedical)				6)		
in business enterprises	−	−	+	p	−	−
in universities	p	+	+	p	−	−
in specialised research centres	p	−	+	p	−	−

Other services (continued)	B	DK	F	G	NL	CH
health administration by						
local/regional authorities						
(municipalities, provinces, etc.)	+	+	+	+	+	+
central government (departments of health)	+	+	+	–	+	+
health insurance boards/bodies/funds	+	o	–	+	+	+
private insurers	+	–	p	+	+	–

Notes

1) Apart from some relics of the health care organisation in the former DDR.

2) Introduced via public nursing care insurance (PNI).

3) Remunerated by private health insurance, given the type of insurance covers such services.

4) Eligible, but no mandatory mass screening.

5) Limited to dental hygiene (no treatment).

6) Still incomplete, because only activities sponsored from public budgets are included.

Annex 2.4: Descriptions of Health Care Concepts

Contents

1. *Health, health care and health care facilities*

1.1. *Health*

Health
A state of complete physical, mental and social well-being and not merely the absence of disease or infirmity.
(WHO)

1.2. *Health care*

Health care
The supply of goods and services in the medical and paramedical field, related to prevention, medical cure (diagnostics and treatment) and paramedical care, provided by trained professionals, institutions and/or companies (or parts of institutions and/or companies) for human beings suffering (or suspected of suffering) from diseases, disabilities and/or limitations of a physical and/or mental nature.
(CvM)

Related issues:

Medical care
Health care provided by qualified physicians with respect to diagnosis, treatment and follow-up of patients. These include: anamnesis (medical history, present problem), physical examination, differential diagnosis and diagnostic planning, requests for medical support, requests for consultation, diagnosis, information and advice to the patient, medication, interventions, referral and discharge, and follow-up.
(SIG)

Nursing care
Health care provided to the patient or individual, assisting him to perform those activities, contributing to health or recovery (or to peaceful decease), which the patient or individual would perform unaided if he would have the required strength, willpower or knowledge. Moreover, nursing care comprises the assistance to the patient in carrying out the treatment plans as prescribed by the responsible health professionals.
Nursing care may be provided by qualified personnel ranging from the nursing aid to the professional nurse and nurse-midwife.
(SIG)

Cure
Emphasis on actions in the (para)medical sphere, aimed at curing and combating diseases.
(CvM)

Care
Emphasis on nursing/caring, aimed at recovery or development of functions, as well as the maintenance of the physical and/or mental condition.
(CvM)

Care of midwives
Care by personnel qualified to guide normal deliveries independently at home, hospitals or maternity clinics.
(CBS)

Maternity care
Family help in case of delivery at home (or in an outpatient department) with special attention for mother and child until about 6 days after birth.
(CBS)

Home help
Services providing housework, such as shopping, cooking, cleaning and administrative work (filling in forms, paying bills). Furthermore the delivery of personal care (help with bathing and dressing) and going for a walk.
(Hutten/Kerkstra)

General medical treatment
Medical treatment given by general practitioners.
(PvS)

General dentistry
Treatment given by dentists, not specialised.
(PvS)

Support of family care
Facilities of a health care institution with the purpose to support members of the family in the care for patients at home.
(PVS)

Support of home care
Facilities of a health care institution with the purpose to support its personnel charged with home care activities.
(PVS)

Holiday relief
Short term admission of a patient motivated by holidays of the usual caretaker(s) at home.
(PVS)

Family care of mental patients
Care for mental patients in a family setting, not being the own family.
(PVS)

Alternative medicine (medical/non medical)
A group of healing techniques and approaches, based on other than scientific medical principles.
(PVS)

Anthroposofic medical treatment
Medical treatment, based on principles as laid down by Rudolf Steiner and his successors.
(PVS)

Intramural care
Health care for patients formally admitted for a period more than 24 hours (intramural) and/or the institutionalised treatment for a substantial part of the day (or night).
(CvM)

Acute care
Establishments receiving patients whose expected average length of stay is less than 30 days.
(OECD)

Long-term care
To refer to the treatment and re-education of individuals with lasting and rehabilitating disabilities in an attempt to restore them as far as possible to their former state of independence and ability to participate in community life.
(SIG)

Extramural care
Health care provided on a non-residential basis, after consultation by the patient delivered by medical and paramedical professionals working from their own premises or co-operating in group practices or health centres and care delivered by organisations, specialised in home care and home nursing.
(CvM)

Out-patient care
Health care provided by specialists, working in out-patient departments of hospitals and using hospital facilities.
(PVS)

Ambulatory care
Sum of extramural care and care by out-patient departments of hospitals.
(PVS)

Total personal health care
Sum of inpatient care, ambulatory care, pharmaceutical consumption and purchased therapeutic appliances.
(OECD)

Preventive care/Prevention
Health care and advice, (usually in general public health programs), aimed at health promotion, the protection of health, preventing the occurrence of diseases or injuries and the early detection of diseases or developmental disorders.
(CvM)

1.3. *Health care facilities*

Health care facility
Institution, company (or part thereof) or practice (combination of self-employed health care professionals and auxiliary personnel) providing services in the health care field.
(CvM)

1.3.1. Intramural health care facilities

Intramural health care facility
Health care facility with accommodation for stay overnight or a substantial part of the day.
(CvM)

Hospital
Intramural health care facility providing medical care and nursing care which consists of observation, diagnosis, therapy and rehabilitation services for persons suffering from a disease or injury or suspected to be suffering from a disease or injury. The hospital may, but needs not, also provide services on an outpatient basis The

hospital may also be a centre for the instruction of health professionals. The hospital may facilitate biomedical and/or social research.
(SIG)

Nursing home
Intramural health care facility providing medical treatment and associated care of people with somatic disabilities and/or psychic disorders, aiming to recover the functions needed in everyday routine and the maintenance of the health status.
(CvM)

Medical children's home
Intramural health care facility for the medical treatment and nursing, including twenty-four hours a day for a limited period of time, of children aged under 16 (except for some special cases), whose physical or mental health is impaired or seriously threatened and for whom at home there is insufficient treatment available, but for whom admission into a hospital or another institution is not or no longer indicated.
(CBS)

Institution for the mentally deficient
Intramural health care facility for the treatment and nursing of persons with (congenital) mental arrears and deficiencies.
(PVS from CBS)

Institution for sensorially handicapped
Intramural health care facility for the deaf and/or partially deaf, or the blind and/or partially blind, which provides social and pedagogic education as well as care, medical treatment (including medical examination), rehabilitation by experts, and nursing, all of this directed towards the ability to receive special education, other education or training as well as possible.
(CBS)

Nursery for toddlers under medical supervision
Intramural health care facility for the medical treatment, nursing and care, in (part of) day time, intended for children aged 1,5 to 6 years (and in some exceptional cases older), whose development is impaired or threatened as a consequence of physical, mental and social circumstances.
(CBS)

Maternity clinic: (specialised hospital)
Intramural health care facility, especially equipped for deliveries with medical indication and postnatal care.
(CvM)

Maternity home
Intramural health care facility, especially equipped for deliveries without medical indication and postnatal care.
(PVS from CBS)

Abortion clinic
Intramural health care facility, predominantly day-care, especially equipped for the termination of pregnancies and related aftercare.
(PVS)

Oncological and radiotherapeutic institute
Intramural health care facility for day care treatment of malignant neoplasm's by radiation and chemotherapy.
(CBS)

Home for the elderly
Residential care facility providing durable lodging, boarding and complete or partial care to persons of 65 years and older.
(PVS from CBS)

Reconvalescence day centres
Intramural health care facility, day care only, providing treatment and care of temporarily or permanently handicapped persons by a team of medical specialists, psychologists and experts in the paramedical. nursing, social, ergonomic and technical field.
(CBS)

Day centre for physically and/or mentally disabled
Intramural health care facility, day care only, providing social and (ped)agogic training with a view to selfmaintenance and integration into society of handicapped persons and providing support and guidance of their social environment.
(PVS from CBS)

Family replacement homes
Intramural health care facility, providing residential accommodation, care and agogic training with a view to independent functioning and selfmaintenance of the handicapped.
(PVS from CBS)

Short term recovery homes
Intramural health care facility providing short term admission, support and nursing care around the clock to patients after medical treatment elsewhere or providing care to patients, normally 16 years and older, with psychosocial problems and

disturbance of daily functioning, for whom ambulatory treatment is not (not yet) sufficient and admission in a psychiatric hospital is not (not yet) necessary.
(PVS from CBS)

Institution for supervised dwelling
Intramural health care facility providing residential accommodation, social training and training in daily functioning and selfmaintenance for patients, who show durable limited social functioning, caused by psychiatric disturbances, and have no sufficiently supporting home environment.
(PVS from CBS)

Health spa
Intramural health care facility providing preventive treatments of various kinds.
(from Brückner)

1.3.2. Extramural health care facilities

Extramural health care facility
Health care facility without accommodation for stay overnight or a substantial part of the day, providing treatment of (physical and mental) diseases by a medical professional and/or (part of) a company).
(CvM)

General Practitioner Practice
Extramural health care facility for the provision of comprehensive medical care as a continuing responsibility regardless of age of the patient or of the condition that may temporarily require the services of a specialist.
(from Dorland)

Group practice
This is a (general) practice of at least three general practitioners with own practices at one and the same address, irrespective of whether they work full-time or part-time. A co-operation of two general practitioners with own practices and one assistant general practitioner is not counted as a group practice.
(CBS)

Specialist practice
Non-institutionalised treatment of (physical and mental) diseases of a specific nature by a (group of) medical specialist(s).
(CVM)

Specialisms supplemented by participants
Specialisms, which are not considered as medical specialisms in the Netherlands, but are added to the list of specialisms by at least one participant
(PvS)

Dental practice
Treatment of patients with diseases affecting their teeth or aberrations in the cavity of the mouth (of a general nature) and the prevention of dental diseases by a dentist (including services by a dental technician or mouth hygienist).
(CvM)

Officinal pharmacy
Extramural health care facility consisting of a room (or rooms) and store-room(s) belonging together, which is/are used by (a) pharmacist(s).
(PVS from CBS)

Blood bank
Extramural health care facility whose main task is the collection of blood (products). The blood bank processes these into blood products and supplies them to hospitals etc. Blood donors donate their blood on a voluntary basis and without payment.
(CBS)

Medical laboratory
Extramural health care facility, sometimes situated in hospitals, serving general practitioners and extramurally working specialists by the examination of materials derived from the human body for the purpose of providing information on diagnosis, prevention, or treatment of diseases.
(PVS from Dorland)

Centre for infants and toddlers
Usually part of a "cross organisation", this is a centre where physicians and nurses provide preventive care for infants and toddlers. Examinations are to a considerable extent aimed at discerning (future) development
disorders.
(CBS)

Institution for ambulatory mental health care
Extramural health care facility aimed at examination and diagnosis, treatment and therapeutic attendance, prevention and guidance of patients/clients with mental and psychosocial problems.
(CVM)

Health centres for alcohol and drug addicts
Institutions providing aid and treatment to alcoholics and drug addicts in the widest sense.
(CBS)

Maternity centre
Extramural health care facility which provides mothers and their new-born babies with home care during the first six days after delivery. This may be on the basis of internal care (in which the maternity aid assists full-time in one family) or district care (in which she assists a family part-time in daily visits). Generally maternity centres are run by the "cross-organisations".
(CBS)

"Cross-organisation" (institutions for domiciliary health and social services)
Extramural health care facility which provide assistance consisting of, among others:
- district nursing: nursing and care of ill and infirm people at home
- centres for infants and toddlers
- giving health information and education
- lending nursing aids and therapeutical appliances
- home help

(from CBS)

Thrombosis service
Extramural health care facility with the task of regularly taking blood samples in order to determine the coagulation time and on this basis indicating the doses of (anti)coagulants.
(CBS)

Health centre
Extramural health care facility of at least one general practitioner with his own practice, one district nurse and one social worker co-operating at one and the same address.
(CBS)

Dispensary
Extramural health care facility where general or specialised medical treatment is provided or preventive activities are deployed concerning e.g. the abatement of TBC, cancer, alcohol abuse and the promotion of food hygiene and sports medicine.
(from CREDES)

Out-patient department
Ambulatory health care facility for specialised consultations an treatment, situated in hospitals and using hospital facilities.
(PVS)

Anti poison centre (for consultation only)
Extramural health care facility, organised as a centre of knowledge and experience concerning the treatment of intoxication's providing consultation services in this field for health care professionals.
(PVS)

Hospital home care
Extramural health care facility of hospitals for care delivery at the patients' home after discharge.
(PVS)

Physical Therapy Practice (Physiotherapy, Cesar, Mensendieck, Ergotherapy)
Extramural health care facility aimed at recovering the functions of the organs of locomotion through different kinds of therapy and/or preventing the further deterioration of the physical functions and increasing the possibilities to function in the living and working environment.
(CvM)

Transport of patients
Transport of patients by ambulance services or other means of transport.
(from CBS)

Ambulance service
Extramural health care facility providing so-called recumbent transport of patients in specially equipped ambulances with specially trained staff. There are two types of transport: emergency transport and ordered transport.
(from CBS)

1.3.3. Preventive health care facilities

Preventive health care facility
Institution providing advice and activities regarding the prevention and early detection of diseases and developmental disorders and the protection of the health status of (groups of) persons as well as health promoting activities to the population.
(CvM)

Municipal Health Service
Preventive health care facility under municipal or intermunicipal authority aimed at promoting the health of the entire population of the municipality(ies) concerned or of specific groups of this population.
(from CBS)

School Health Service
An institution for diagnostic and preventive care of school aged children by special public health physicians.
(from CBS)

School dental service
An institution for diagnostic, preservative and preventive dental care of children at nursery and primary schools.
(CBS)

Occupational health service
An institution which aims to watch over the health status of the employees of one or more enterprises and to protect them against injurious influences of their work.
(CBS)

1.3.4. Other services

The group of "other services" is described as a rest category of provisions with three circumscribed sets of activities:
- education and training of health care staff
- health research and development
- administration

Research & development
Research and development is divided in a part on biomedics and a part on pharmaceuticals.
Biomedical research comprises the study of specific diseases, including the treatment thereof and rehabilitation; the design of methods, drugs and devices used in the aforementioned process; and finally the scientific investigations in this field leading to new methods, procedures, solutions, etc.
Pharmaceutical research comprises all activities carried out in the enterprise sector.
(OECD Health data bank 1997)

Education & Training
Number of students enrolled in paramedical schools, undergraduate schools in medical/biomedical departments and graduate schools in medical/biomedical departments.
It would also include health education reported by local and central authorities for the training of health workers.

Complete expenditures would include universities and other training institutions. Salaries of medical interns, nurse trainees are included in the expenditures of the institutions, not as training expenditures.
(OECD Health data bank 1997)

Administration
Expenditures by private insurers and by central and local authorities including health insurance boards and health boards delivering medical care for planning, management, regulation, fund collecting, handling of claims of the delivery system and other administrative bodies.
Administrative costs born by the providers (such as patient records and hospital management) are not included in general administration.
(OECD Health data bank 1997)

1.3.5. Medical goods

Medical goods
Pharmaceuticals, wound dressings and bandages, and therapeutic appliances.
(CVM)

1.3.5.1. Pharmaceuticals

Pharmaceutical
Medicinal substance or agent
(Dorland's Illustrated Medical Dictionary, Philadelphia, 1988)

Wound dressing
Any of various materials utilised for covering and protecting a wound.
(Dorland's Illustrated Medical Dictionary, Philadelphia, 1988)

Bandage
Strip or roll of gauze or other material for wrapping or binding any part of the body.
(Dorland's Illustrated Medical Dictionary, Philadelphia, 1988)

Total expenditure on pharmaceuticals
The consumption of pharmaceutical products includes prescriptions and self-medication, often referred to as over-the-counter (OTC) products. The series includes the pharmacists' remuneration when the latter is separate from the price of medicines. Pharmaceuticals consumed in hospitals are excluded. The expenditures includes VAT and sales taxes where applicable. The value of consumption in hospitals is included under in-patient care.
(OECD)

– *with prescription*
Expenditure on medicines, exclusively sold to customers with a medical prescription.
(OECD)

– *without prescription*
Expenditure on medicines that do not need a prescription, often called Over-The Counter.
(OECD)

1.3.5.2. Therapeutic appliances

Therapeutic appliance
Any device, apparatus or instrument for performing or facilitating the performance of a particular physical function in a desired way or for disguising the absence or bad operation of that function.
(PVS to Dorland's Illustrated Medical Dictionary, Philadelphia, 1988)

Total expenditures on therapeutic appliances
Expenditure on therapeutic appliances and materials (e.g. optical equipment, hearing devices, wheelchairs), excluding appliances supplied in hospitals.
Excludes Medical Prosthesis
Excludes Dental Prosthesis
The expenditures listed include VAT and sales taxes where applicable.
(OECD)

2. *Health care professions*

Health care employment
Number of persons employed (sometimes expressed in full-time equivalent persons) in health-related activities, including external personnel under contract, not including employment in the pharmaceutical and medical equipment industry. Administrative staff and personnel employed by private and non-profit health insurance are included. Health professionals working in non-health related industries are excluded. Conversions in full-time equivalent vary between countries; they are often made on the basis of a 35 hour workweek at the minimum.
(OECD)

Health Professional
Any health care worker with full professional qualifications (according to WHO or similar standards) who is qualified and capable to care for those suffering from or

affected by disease, to prevent disease and/or to promote community and/or individual health.
(SIG)

Physician
A person who, having been regularly admitted to a medical school, duly recognised in the country where it is located, has successfully completed the prescribed course of studies in medicine, and who has acquired the
requisite qualifications to be legally licensed to practice medicine (comprising prevention, diagnosis, treatment and rehabilitation) using independent judgement, to promote individual and community health.
(Official Records of WHO, 1972 no. 198, pages 14, 80–81; No. 201, page 20)
(SIG)

Active physicians
Number of physicians (general practitioners and specialists/consultants), not including qualified physicians working abroad, but including foreign physicians authorised to practice in the country
(OECD)

Nurse
A health professional who has the qualifications and authorisations (possibly country-specific) or is in training to supply the nursing care for the care of patients, the promotion of health and the prevention of illness and to support physicians and other health professionals in carrying out the diagnostic, therapeutic and follow-up plans for the benefit of the patient, by informing, supporting and assisting them.
(SIG)

Paramedical professions
This group includes, in a strict sense, approved non-medical specialists designated as such, who support and complement the therapeutic activities of medical practitioners. The following professions were approved: physical therapists, exercise therapists Mensendieck and Cesar, dieticians, orthopticians, oral hygienists, radiographers, speech therapists, occupational therapists, chiropodists.
In a wider sense, the paramedical professions also cover those of a medical-technical and medical assistance rendering nature which provide, on the basis of a less scientifically accentuated training, support and assistance in medical activities (laboratory assistants, opticians, instrument makers, dental technicians etc.).
(CBS)

Specialist physician
A physician who has received special training in one branch of medicine, and who limits his practice, in whole or in part, to particular disease categories or to certain

age groups. A specialist physician's work is concerned, in whole or in part, with patients that have been referred by other physicians.
(SIG)

General practitioner
A physician, authorised to provide comprehensive medical care as a continuing responsibility regardless of age of the patient or of the condition that may temporarily require the services of a specialist
(from Dorland)

Dentist
A person who has received a degree from an accredited school of dentistry and is licensed to practice dentistry by a state board of dental examiners.
(Dorland)

Pharmacist
One who is licensed to prepare and sell or dispense drugs and compounds, and to make up prescriptions and who is responsible for medication surveillance, consultancy of prescriptors and information to patients.
(Dorland/NRV)

Druggist
Druggist (drogisten) are allowed to sell a limited number of pharmaceutical specialities and preparations, which may be sold without prescription and which are not exclusively reserved for pharmacies.
(CBS)

Midwife
A midwife is entitled to advice pregnant women, to conduct normal deliveries independently or under the responsibility of a practising physician, to take blood or material for cytostatical preparations, to conduct epitosomias with application of local anaesthesia and to stitch lacerations of limited size.
(from NRV)

Maternity home helps
Specially trained workers who take care of mother and child, at home, following the delivery. This work is included in the home care services rendered by the "cross-organisations".
(CBS)

Physiotherapist
Applies, after referral by a practising physician, one or more of the following therapies: movement therapy, massage therapy and physical therapy in a strict sense i.e. the application of physical stimuli electrotherapy, ultra-sound therapy,

thermotherapy, hydrotherapy, balneotherapy and electrodiagnostics, with the exclusion of the application of ionising beams.
(PVS from NRV)

Ergotherapist
observes, after referral by a practising physician, impediments in daily activities and labour, trains patients in dealing with these impediments, whether or not with application of expedients, and advises patients with regard to living and work conditions and provisions needed.
(PVS from Dorland)

Podiatrist (chiropodist)
a specialist in podiatry (the specialised field that deals with the study and care of the foot, including its anatomy, pathology, medical and surgical treatment.
(Dorland)

Speech therapist
examines speech defects under the responsibility of a practising physician or dentist and improves speech abilities of patients by relief of deficiencies or breath regulation.
(from NRV)

Dental hygienist
examines teeth under responsibility of a practising dentist and reports about dental conditions and surrounding tissues, cleans teeth, applies preserving and preventing means at teeth and surrounding tissues and informs patients with regard to dental hygiene behaviour.
(from NRV)

Dental prothetist
fits and manufactures complete dentures for edentulous patients (without dental elements left).
(from NRV)

Dental technician
Manufactures, by order of dentist or orthodontist, dentures, crowns, jackets, regulation plates and the like.
(from NRV)

Orthoptist
An expert in orthoptics (a technique of eye exercises designed to correct the visual axis of eyes properly co-ordinated for binocular vision).
(Dorland)

Podotherapist
applies, after referral by a practising physician, corrective and protective therapies concerning foot functions, treats external defects of the skin of the foot and prevents and treats nail defects.
(from NRV)

Psychotherapist
examines and treats patients with mental disorders or complaints by application of professional methods in order to influence frame of mind, behaviour and attitudes.
(from NRV)

Dietician
composes diets adjusted to patients for medical purposes under the responsibility of a physician or dentist and advises patients with regard to their diet.
(from NRV)

Medical analyst
examines for diagnostic purposes, by order of a physician, patient material (liquids, tissues, excrement's) by means of chemical, immunological, haematological, microbiological, histological, cytological and nuclear technics.
(from NRV)

Sources

CBS: Compendium of Health Statistics 1986, The Hague, 1986
Health, United States, 1991: Appendix II "Glossary"
OECD: OECD Health Systems; Facts and Trends 1960–1991, Paris, 1993
OECD: OECD Health data bank 1997
GSS Government Statistical Service: "Health and Personal Services Statistics for England, 1992 edition", London, 1993.
SIG: "The emerging ENS Care Statistics distributed database"; Definitions, Classifications and conversions for hospital data by Hospital Statistics Working Group, compiled by SIG Services, Netherlands, 1993.
WHO, 1977: "World Health Annual Statistics 1977", Genève
BASYS: Schneider c.s., "Gesundheitssysteme im Internationalen Vergleich, Ausgabe 1992", BASYS, Augsburg, 1993
Dorland's illustrated Medical Dictionary 27th Edition, Philadelphia, 1985
"Beroepengids Zorgsector", Nationale Raad voor de Volksgezondheid, Zoetermeer, 1990
CvM: C. van Mosseveld, "Health Care: Concepts & Classifications", Voorburg, 1988 (unpublished document).
PVS: P. van Son

Annex 2.5: Leading papers pepared for the first Consultation of the Network of Experts, Voorburg, 21–23 September 1994

Revised version, 30-3-1995

Authors:

Dr. M. Schneider:
" Framework for international comparison of health expenditures and financing"

Dr. S. Sandier:
"Problems regarding manpower in international comparison"

J.-P. Poullier:
"Inputs and throughputs in in-patient care"

C.J.P.M. van Mosseveld / J.M. Smit:
"Data on supply of health care"

International Comparison of Health Systems
Framework for international comparison of health expenditures and financing

Discussion Paper

Markus Schneider

January 1995
BASYS, D-86159 Augsburg, Reisingerstr. 25, Tel.: +49-821-257940
Fax: +49-821-579341

1. *Introduction*

Health expenditures are not compiled in a uniform way in the European Communities. Not only the conventional definitions vary but also the classification. Therefore, international comparisons of the scope and structure of health sector are only possible by adjustments of national figures to an uniform concept [1)]. These adjustments are often based on rough estimations and cannot replace exact compilations by common definitions.

There are two problems on the way to a uniform health care expenditure statistics in the European Union

1. The concept of health expenditure accounting should be identical within the Member States
2. The concept should be used in the same way.

Presently, health care expenditures are computed in the European Union within the national statistical offices on different concepts. Some countries use the concept of final consumption of medical services and goods within the framework of the Systems of National Accounts (SNA). This is the concept of the OECD, which is the leading concept within the European Union used by health economists and in health policy (see appendix D). The concept is used in a different classification of services and goods by some Member States, e.g. by Dutch Statistical Office (see appendix C) or by the French Statistical Office for accounting "La consommation médicale totale" (see appendix A).

A different approach is used by EUROSTAT based on the European systematic of social protection (ESSPROS). This concept starts from the risks which should be covered under public social protection schemes. Although ESSPROS contains both benefits in kind and cash benefits it differs systematically from the two former concepts, because it is primarily directed to the compilation of the public transfers in the case of sickness (see appendix E) [2)]. A mixed concept between the SNA approach and ESSPROS is used by the German Statistical Office "Ausgaben für Gesundheit". This approach goes beyond the NA-concept because beyond medical consumption additionally cash benefits for health are included (see appendix B), it goes beyond ESSPROS because private insurance is included.

Based on the national institutional framework of organizing health protection and health care the used concepts vary in all Member States. An overview gives table 1. Furthermore, the definition of the boundaries of the health sector within the economy vary. Also, the terminology is different (see annexes). For example, the Dutch accounting system is called „Costs and Financing of Health Care", the French system „National Accounts of Health", the German system „Expenditures for Health".

Besides, in the definition of health services often a mix between kind of expenditure and sector delivered is used.

All national accounts do not include activities of household production of health as home care by family members or activities for regeneration. Furthermore, it has to be considered that the national statistics do not contain information on the utilization of services by different socioeconomic groups.

Table 1:
Concepts of health expenditure accounting used by the Member States

Country	Main Concept	Remarks
Belgium	SNA	Different use of private/public consumption in the national accounts, no research and development, and education
Danmark	Nordic concept	Similarities to ESSPROS, nursing homes not included
France	SNA	Detailed Computations for the financing side
Germany	Mixed SNA, ESSPROS	Including cash benefits, no private expenditures for nursing homes
Greece	E, SNA	No research and development, and education, nursing homes not included
Italy	E, SNA	No research and development, and education, nursing homes not included
Ireland	SNA	No research and development, and education
Luxemburg	E	No research and development, and education, nursing homes not included
Netherlands	SNA	No research and development, and education
Portugal	E	No research and development, and education, nursing homes not included
Spain	E	No research and development, and education, nursing homes not included
United Kingdom	SNA	No research and development, and education, nursing homes not included

SNA = National Accounts, E = ESSPROS.

The main shortage of all concepts is that they are not applied in a uniform way by the Member States. But this does not result from the definitions or the concept per se rather from applying the guidelines to use the concept as well as from weak interests of national authorities to support the concept. The major disadvantage from the viewpoint of policy analysis are presently the limited possibilities to compare the service sectors as well as to split policy areas as prevention, care, or rehabilitation. Especially, health expenditure accounting offers only a limited classification to analyze the activities in the Member States in the field of health protection. Also on the financing side a more detailed classification of sources of funds would be desirable.

2. *Steps to a common concept*

All concepts requires some compromises. It must be defined which activities and goods should be included, what should be excluded. Prerequisite is a clear definition what is the purpose of the concept. There are four main objectives

1. The concept should help the national health policy in the resource allocation and distribution process
2. The concept should help to support the health protection policy of the EU
3. The concept should show flows of medical services and goods among Member States
4. The concept should allow international comparisons among the developed countries.

The OECD choice of the conceptual framework have been dictated by two practical considerations: [3)]

a. the concept should be part of a wider analysis of social policies and their interrelatedness with economic policies (the natural link being the use of a common macro-accounting framework),

b. SNA and ESA already offer a large body of ground rules and definitions common to all OECD Member countries, and an incomplete but existing reporting mechanism around which to build the aggregates wanted.

Accounting of health care expenditures and financing is not a goal in itself but derived as mean to inform of allocation and distribution of health expenditures and financing. Therefore, the applied theoretical approach is essential for compilation and outcome. In general, the following questions have to be answered by health accounting.

- How are expenditures distributed according to the type of services delivered and involved production units?
- What is the output of the health system and what is the share of the gross domestic health product on the total gross domestic product?
- Which share of the national health expenditures is spent for public health, activities as compared with health care?
- What are the costs of the health system?
- How are services and producing units of the health systems financed by financial institutions via private and public means?

Because of different institutional frameworks of the health systems in the Member States as well as different focal points of health policies the national requests on the health expenditure data vary. Health expenditures statistics are derived more by existing institutional conditions than by common conceptual ideas. The demand for international comparability has therefore to concentrate on the basic figures of the health system. But, what are basic figures?

Without going too much into details basic figures should inform about the total and the structure of production, consumption and financing as well as the margins.

Therefore, to reach international comparability first and foremost the applied definition of the total and its break down has to be the same for all countries of the analysis. Furthermore, a common accounting methodolgy should be used.
Health expenditure statistics based on the framework of the national accounts may be handled as satellite system. The reference to the System of National Accounts is a conditio sine qua non. However, satellite systems do not always imply a full integration of the health care sector. For example, factor incomes are often not computed by different health care sectors. It would be useful to have a full descripton of health expenditure compilation in all Member States.
Independently of the applied concept aggreement should be reached with respect to a uniform classification of the expenditure and financing side of health protection expenditures and health care expenditures. Both sides should be classified in a more detailed way as in the present classification of the OECD-Concept.

- It is necessary to discuss the split between
- health protection and health care
- consumption and investment
- research and education
- benefits in kind and cash benefits
- sectors and services
- wages and other factor costs
- public and private financing institutions
- extramural and intramural institutions
- expenditures to current and constant prices.

It is proposed to discuss in a second step in detail what problems will arise if the concept will be applied to certain Member States. The concept should be proved in collaboration with National Statistical Offices. The problems should be documented. Based on the common definitions and the documented problems a manual should be developed that can be used to compute the health expenditures in a standardized way. [4]

3. *Health production and health goods and services*

As mentioned above, different approaches are possible in the compilation of health expenditures. From the viewpoint of health economics the relation to health production is essential. Therefore, in the following only two approaches will be distinguished:

1. the health production approach (total income approach)
2. the health goods and services approach (SNA-approach)

The first approach starts from the assumption that health is produced by indivduals and consumption of health care goods delivered by hospitals and physiciancs are intermediate consumption in the household production of health. The output in this approach is measured by the valued total time of the household spending for health

production plus the consumption of health services and goods produced by private and public enterprises.
In the second approach household production plays only a marginal role. Instead, it focuses on the production of health care services in markets and by government institutions. This traditional approach is widedly realized by the System of National Accounts). It is used in mainstream economics, by the OECD and by several statistical offices as basis for health expenditure accounting. Nevertheless, this approach is not satisfactory from the viewpoint of health economics.
The same holds true for the welfare or tranfer approach used by EUROSTAT. This approach looks on the health transfers in kind and health transfers in cash delivered to households. It focuses on the social proctecion of households. Private protection is excluded.

The health production approach as well as the health goods and services approach is linked to the System of National Accounts (SNA). The SNA consists of a coherent, consistent and integrated set of macroeconomic accounts, balance sheets and tables based on a set of internationally agreed concepts, definitions, classifications and accounting rules. In general, the accounting of the health system does not use the complete set of tables of the SNA. Accumulation accounts and balance sheets are not used. Besides, some assumptions are introduced, e.g. not to account the relation to the rest of the world or changes of inventories.
In the center of the health expenditure compilations is the assumption that the following equation holds:
production of health care = consumption of health care = costs of health care = income from health care.

Using this equation, in practise, some additional terms have to be considered as intermediate consumption, capital formation, changes of inventories (see table 1). A further problem is that several producing units exist with heterogeneous production structures. The same is true on the financing side. Therefore, the identification and classification of health activities within all producing units of a country are major challenges. The identification of activities of several ambulatory and institutional health producing units is a necessary step to develop a common classification.
The economic analysis of production is mainly concerned with activities that produce outputs of a kind that can be delivered or provided to other institutional units. Unless outputs are produced which can be supplied to other units, either individually or collectively, there can be no division of labour, no specialization of production and no gains from trading. In order to be able to delineate activities that are productive in an economic sense from other activities, it is necessary to define the characteristics of both *goods* and *services* which are the two main kinds of outputs. Given the general characteristics of the goods and services produced as outputs, it becomes possible to define production.

Table 2
Production account: Value added/Gross Domestic Product

Production	Consumption	Costs
Output Intermediate consumption (–) Indirect taxes, less subsidies	Final Consumption Changes in inventories Gross fixed capital formation Acquisitions less disposals Exports less imports	Compensation of Employees Taxes on production and imports Subsidies (–) Operating surplus/mixed income
GDP Consumption of fixed capital NDP	GDP	GDP

In the SNA the intermediate inputs are recorded and valued at the time they enter the production process, while outputs are recorded and valued as they emerge from the process. Intermediate inputs are normally valued at purchasers´ prices and outputs as basic prices or alternatively at producers´ prices, if basic prices are not available. In the context of the production account, the output consists only of those goods and services which are produced within establishments being available for use outside these establishments. In practise, some of the goods sold or otherwise used within any given accounting period may have been withdrawn from inventiories of goods produced in previous periods.
In the most countries health accounting does not consider the accumulation of capital. This major shortfall of health accounting is especially true in the field of human capital. Expenditures for R&D and for education of health staff is part of the human capital formation of a country.

4. *Boundaries of the health system*

As mentioned above the compilation of health goods and services consumed or produced requires are clear definition of these goods and services. The definition of health services and goods is the starting point for all further definitions.
If we started instead with the definition of the producing units the boundaries of the health system would have to be drawn from the other sectors of economy. Starting from goods and services on the one hand and producing units on the other hand will not automatically lead to the same result. Producing units may produce various types of goods and services. Only those activities have to be accounted which are by definition part of the health system. Therefore, on the institutional side we have to group producing units most homogeneously after the clarification of the goods and services which are part of the health sector. Producing units which only partly produce health goods should also be included; for example, old-age-homes should only be part of the health system with their long-term care activities.
Often, in health accounting the output of producing units is regarded as homogenous. For example, hospitals produce inpatient services. If this was true, then the structure of expenditures or activities could be compiled without detailed analysing the interconnection of producing units and services. But, if this assumption

does not hold, then the compilation of a matrix between the kind of delivered health services and the type of producing units is essential to understand the differences in production of health services and goods.

The interconnection is shown in table 4. The matrix has three dimensions: the activities, the producing units and the technology (with beds or no beds). [5)]

Health goods and services are in the definition of the classification of goods of the national accounts; such goods are primarily produced for health purposes. In the national accounts only those goods are considered, which are produced by private and public institutions for money. This definition includes the so-called public goods which can be consumed simultaneously by all persons such as the control of water or the reduction of infections by vaccinations.

Table 3
Health production by goods and producing units

	Public Health producing units	Extramural producing units	Intramural producing units	Other producing units	Private Households	Rest of the world
Public Health						
Occupational health						
School health						
Maternity						
Screening						
Others						
Health Care						
Medical Care						
no beds						
with beds						
Dental Care						
no beds						
with beds						
Paramedical Care						
no beds						
with beds						
Long-term care						
no beds						
with beds						
Ambulances						
Other services						
Drugs						
Medical aids						
Others						
Administration						
Total 1						
Education						
R&D						
Capital formation						
Total 2						

Health goods which are delivered freely by non-profit-institutions are also included. Not included are products produced by households as the care for sick children. Household production is considered insofar as housemaids are paid or as it contains the consumption of health goods produced by public and private institutions. This point is not satisfactory because also unpaid health activities of household members basically support the health production by individuals. Therefore, the total income approach includes the unpaid care of family members. [6]

For the classification of health goods the International Standard Industrial Classifications of All Economic Activities (ISIC) as well as the Central Product Classification (CPC) are not sufficient. A common used international classifcation of health goods and services does not exist. The international classification of medical procedures (ICPM) does not contain all health goods and is not yet applied by the Member States. Nevertheless, a complete classification of the services has to be developed. One criterion for including a service in the list is the ability of substitution by other services.

Beside the production boundary the national boundary has to be considered. Not all health goods produced within the borders of a country are consumed by the population of the country. Presently, the cross-country flows of health services are very low, but not that of health goods as pharmaceuticals or medical equipment. The consideration of these international trade effects would be desirable [7].
In the discussion of the costs of health systems, costs and expenditures are often used as synonyms, although the meaning is different. [8] Costs result from the production of health goods. Costs are related directly to the production process contrary to expenditures which measure the flow of liquidity. [9] Also, the classification of costs differ from the classification of expenditures.
Health services and goods should be split in two broad categories public health and health care because the nature of the products vary as well as the production process.

5. *Financing health goods and services*

Differences in the published financing structures of the health system result mainly from differences of the boundaries of the health systems. The common boundaries of health services of goods are therefore prerequisite for the compilation of the financing side. Health accounting often starts from the funding institutions (government, social security, private insurance, enterprises, private households) because on this level the best statistics are available and many payments to producing units are not for specific services (see table 4). If, for example, outpatient and inpatient services of households are paid by a common budget, then, in general, the statistics of inpatient and outpatient are not available.
More of interest are the questions which health serives and goods are financed by which agents (see table 5). Prerequisite for the compilation of this table is table 3.

Table 4
Financing of health production

Funding units	Producing units					
	Public Health producing units	Extramural producing units	Intramural producing units	Others	Households	Rest of the world
Government						
Social security						
Private Insurance						
Companies						
Private Households						
Others						
Total						
Balance						

Table 5
Financing of health goods and services

	Government	Social security	Private Enterprises	Others	Households
Public Health					
Occupational health					
School health					
Maternity					
Screening					
Others					
Health Care					
Medical Care					
Dental Care					
Paramedical Care					
Longterm care					
Ambulances					
Other services					
Drugs					
Medical aids					
Other goods					
Administration					
Total 1					
Education					
R&D					
Capital formation					
Total 2					

The account of financing of health goods includes two parts, the funding of the institutions which pay for health goods and services by taxes, contribution etc. (funding process) and the payment of these institutions for the delivering health goods by captitation, fee-for-services, budgets etc. (payment process). The first part is accounted on the revenue side, the latter on the expenditure side of the income account.

The identification of the ultimate bearer of the expenses is not always obvious. In the satellite accounts of SNA the following classification of ultimate financing units is used: (a) Market producers; (b) NPISHs; (c) General Government; (d) Households; (e) Financial Enterprises; (f) Rest of the world. [10] In accounting of the health system the interconnection of financing units is of special interest. Social security and private insurance are then secondary financing units.

6. *Conclusions*

This paper deals only with some aspects of the international comparison of health expenditure and financing. I have not discussed the accumulation of capital, internal trade and prices as well as cash benefits and manpower.

The paper proposes four steps to improve comparability:

1. The definition of the boundary of the health system by the delivered health goods and services has to be the first step of international comparison.
2. For the selected health services and goods the output of all producing units has to be compiled. The interconnection of producing units and health goods and services should be presented in a matrix (goods x productions units x technology).
3. Expenditures for R&D, education and capital formation may be neglected in the short run but in the long run they should be compiled in connection with the accumulation accounts and balance sheets.
4. Unpaid household production in the form of health care for familiy members should be added to the computation of production of health goods and services.

Notes

[1] See OECD (1993), OECD Health Systems: Facts and Trends 1960-1991, Volume I, OECD Health Systems: The Socio-economic Environment, Statistical References, Volume II, Paris; Schneider M et. al. (1993), Gesundheitssysteme im internationalen Vergleich, Augsburg: BASYS, Rublee DA, Schneider M (1991), International Health Spending: Comparison with the OECD, in: Health Affairs, Fall 1991:187-198; Schieber GJ, Poulier J-P (1991), Advancing the debate on international spending comparisons, in Health Affairs, Fall 1991: 199-201.

[2] See Eurostat (1994), Recueil statistique sur la protection sociale en Europe, Tome 5 - Maladie, Luxembourg.

[3] OECD (1985), Measuring health Care 1960–1985, Expenditure, Costs and Performance, Paris.

[4] For the measurement of scientific and technical activities the OECD has developed the so-called "Frascati Manual", Paris 1993.

[5] For semimural care additional lines may be introduced. An alternative approach is to distinguish between first-line and second-line providers, see Hurst Jeremy, The Reform of Health Care. A comparative Analysis of Seven OECD Countries, Paris 1992

[6] Not all kinds of unpaid housework will be included as washing or cleaning. Only those services will be included which may be replaced by market services, see Eisner R., The total incomes system of accounts, The University of Chicago Press, Chicago 1989.

[7] Hermesse Jean, Lewalle Henri, L´accès aux soins en Europe. Quelle mobilité du patient?, Louvain-la-Neuve 1993.

[8] See e.g. Kauling R.H.C.M. , Oosterhof W.G., Health Accounts: An Approach to an Infrastructure, in: Levy E., Accounting for health: An International Survey, Economica, Paris 1982, pp 41–54.

[9] Van Sluijs A., Jansen R., Kosteninformatie in R.M.Lapre en F.F.H. Rutten, Economie van de gezondheitszorg, De Tijdstroom, Lochem 1988, pp. 244–264.

[10] See *Inter-Secretariat Working Group on National Accounts*: Systems of National Accounts 1993, Zif. 21.87.

Appendix A: The French "Comptes Nationaux de la Santé"

The French health accounting system computes two main aggregates:
La consommation médicale totale et la dépense courante de santé.

La consommation médicale totale

- La consommation de soins et de biens medicaux
  1. Soins hospitaliers & en sections médicalisées
     11. Soins hospitaliers
     12. Soins on section médicalisées
  2. Soins ambulatoires
     21. Médecines
     22. Auxiliaires médicaux
     23. Dentists
     24. Analyses
     25. Cure Thermales
  3. Transports de malades
  4. Médicaments
  5. Prothèses
- La consommation de services de médecine préventive
  1. Les services de médecine du travail
  2. Les services de médecine scolaire
  3. La protection maternelle et infantile
  4. Les autres service sanitaires de prévention individualisés (maladies mentales, toxicomanie, alcoolisme...)

La Dépense courante de santé

- Dépenses pour les malades
  1. Soins et biens médicaux
  2. Aide aux malades
  3. Subventions au système de soins
- Dépenses de Prévention
- Dépenses en faveur du systeme de soins
  1. Recherche médicale et pharmaceutique
  2. Formation
- Dépense de Gestion Générale
- Double Compte

Appendix B: The German "Ausgaben für Gesundheit"

Leistungsarten im Gesundheitsbereich (Statistisches Bundesamt)

1.	Vorbeugende und betreuende Maßnahmen
1.1	Gesundheitsdienste
1.2	Gesundheitsvorsorge und Früherkennung (soweit nicht 1.1)
1.3	Betreuende Maßnahmen (soweit nicht 1.1)
1.3.1	Mutterschaftshilfe
1.3.2	Maßnahmen zur Pflege
2.	Behandlung
2.1	Ambulante Behandlung
2.2	Stationäre Behandlung
2.3	Stationäre Kurbehandlung
2.4	Arzneien, Heil- und Hilfsmittel, Zahnersatz
2.4.1	Arzneien, Heil- und Hilfsmittel
2.4.2	Zahnersatz
3.	Krankheitsfolgeleistungen
3.1	Berufliche und soziale Rehabilitation
3.1.1	Berufliche Rehabilitation
3.1.2	Soziale Rehabilitation
3.2	Maßnahmen zur Sicherung des Lebensunterhaltes bei Krankheit und Invalidität
3.2.1	Entgeltfortzahlung
3.2.2	Sonstige Einkommensleistungen im Krankheitsfall
3.2.3	Berufs- und Erwerbsunfähigkeitsrenten
3.3	Sonstige Krankheitsfolgen
4.	Ausbildung und Forschung
4.1	Ausbildung von medizinischem Personal, medizinische Forschung an Hochschulen
4.2	Forschung außerhalb von Hochschulen
5.	Nicht aufteilbare Ausgaben

Quelle: Statistisches Bundesamt 1978.

Appendix C: Dutch Health Expenditure Classification

There are two concepts in the Netherlands: The concept of the Centraal Bureau voor de Statistiek and the Concept of the Tweede Kamer. The Concept of the Centraal Bureau voor de Statistiek is described as follows:

1. Instellingen voor intramurale gezondheidszorg
   - 1.1 Ziekenhuizen
   - 1.2 Psychiatrische Ziekenhuizen
   - 1.3 Inrichtingen voor zwakzinnigen
   - 1.4 Verpleeghuizen
   - 1.5 Andere intramurale instellingen
2. Instellingen en praktijken voor extramurale gezondheidszorg
   - 2.1 Specialistenpraktijken
   - 2.2 Huisartsenpraktiijken
   - 2.3 Instellingen en praktijken voor tandheelkundige hulp
   - 2.4 Praktijken van verloskundigen en paramedici
   - 2.5 Leveranciers van genees- en verbandmiddelen enz.
   - 2.6 Instellingen voor maatschappelijke gezondheitszorg
   - 2.7 Andere extramurale instellingen
3. Instellingen voor overige gezondheidszorg
   - 3.1 Keuringsdiensten voor voedsel en drinkwater
   - 3.2 Beleid, administratie en beheer

Source: CBS, kosten en financiering van de gezondheidszorg 1992.

Appendix D: The OECD Classification

D.1
Expenditures

Total expenditure on health	Public expenditure on health
Total investment on health	Public investment on health
Total expenditure on health administration	Public expenditure on health administration
Total expenditure on biomedical R&D	Public expenditure on biomedical R&D
	Expenditure on armed forces health services
	Expenditure on school health services
	Expenditure on prison health services
	Expenditure on industrial medicine
Total medical consumption – Personal health services	Public medical consumption – Personal health services
Total expenditure on inpatient care	Public expenditure on inpatient care
Total expenditure on acute hospital care	Public expenditure on acute hospital care
Total expenditure on psychiatric hospital care	Public expenditure on psychiatric hospital care
Total expenditure on nursing home care	Public expenditure on nursing home care
Total expenditure on ambulatory medical services	Public expenditure on ambulatory medical services
Total expenditure on physician services	Public expenditure on physician services
Total expenditure on dental services	Public expenditure on dental services
Total expenditure on laboratory tests	Public expenditure on laboratory tests
Total expenditure on x- rays & imaging diagnostics	Public expenditure on x- rays & imaging diagnostics
Total expenditure on pharmaceutical goods	Public expenditure on pharmaceutical goods
Total expenditure on therapeutic appliances	Public expenditure on therapeutic appliances

D.2
Prices

Implicit price indices for medical care & health services
Implicit price indices for medical care private consumption
Implicit price indices for general government price services
Implicit price indices for in-patient care
Implicit price indices for acute hospital care
Implicit price indices for ambulatory care
Implicit price indices for physician services
Implicit price indices for dental services
Implicit price indices for pharmaceutical consumption
Implicit price indices for medical care & health services

Appendix E: Fonction Maladie (Méthodologie SESPROS)

1 Regimes de Base
- 10 *Prestations en espèces*
  - 11 Maintien du salaire
    - A. par l'employeur
    - B. par l'institution de sécuriteé sociale
  - 13 Autres prestation en espèces
  - 14 Données non disponibles par types de prestations
- 20 *Prestations en nature*
  - 21 Hospitalisation
  - 22 Soins ambulatoires
  - 23 Produits pharmaceutiques
  - 24 Soins dentaires
  - 25 Prothèses médicales
  - 26 Analyses médicales et autres examens
  - 27 Prévention
  - 28 Autres prestations en nature
  - 29 Données non disponibles par type de prestations

2 Regimes complementaires

3 Regimes sous conditions de ressources

Problems regarding manpower in international comparison [1)]

Simone Sandier
Research Director
CREDES, Paris

Introduction

Generally production and distribution of goods and services require the combined functioning of production factors: personnel and material. In the health care sector, principally in the services sector, the role of personnel is extremely important. From the economic point of view one might say, that the main part (about 80%) of health care expenditures are attributed to the remuneration of personnel and that the health care sector, especially since the end of the second world war, employs an important part of the active population, which, of course with national variations, is estmimated at 7 to 8%.

The number of people employed in the production and administration of services, their training in different qualifications, their working conditions, their productivity and their economic position constitute important parameters, by which we can learn a lot in international comparison.

The goal of this paper is to review the characteristics, that have to be taken into account when describing capacity and activities of the manpower, employed in the health care sector, and to enumerate the corresponding elements, which might serve as a base for internationally comparative tables. The subjects, treated in this paper, are not exhaustive and probably do not apply to all countries. The choice has been influenced by the French case and by the lack of experience of the author with statistics in other countries. They are ubject to discussion and comments will be welcomed.

General remarks on the parameters to be taken into account when des cribing manpower in health care

Generally spoken countries annually publish statistics on the numbers of personnel, employed in the health care sector. These statistics mostly have been established by the Health Ministries, which execute general control of the system or by social security organizations, which contract the health professionals.

These usually available statistics indicate the capacity, taking into account, on a more or less detailed level, the professional qualifications (physicians, pharmacists, nurses) and the working places (hospitals, health centres, private practices). Moreover, these statistics sometimes comprise, in a less systematic way, the demographic structure of the different professions, their sub-specialties (for example medical specialisms, general nurses, psychiatric nurses), their full-time or part time employment and their remunerations.

Qualifications

One has to be sure, that with the same term, for example "physician", through all countries, persons are indicated, who have received equivalent professional training and who fulfil analogous functions. First criterion is the **certificate**, that must be acquired as a condition for practice in different professions.

Professional training generally is assured and warranted by governmental power in relation with health care institutions, public or private. However, the content of the training programme and the quality of training hardly can be evaluated, but the number of years of training after secondary education, necessary for certification, is a quantitative variable, that all countries can describe. In certain cases it will be possible to indicate more precisely the division of study duration in theoretical studies and practical periods, in which students are working in health care and are charged with certain responsibilities. The conditions of certification may be specified in terms of variants in each category (for example generalists versus specialists).

Place of work

Health care professionals work either in health care institutions, either individually in own premises (for example general paractitioners' office). In the former case professionals of different qualifications are grouped together in cooperation for the distribution of services in favor of the patients of these institutions. This of course applies to hospital institutions, but also applies to the case of health centres and sometimes to the case of group practices.

Personnel not only comprises medical professions, but also technical personnel (for example engineers and radiological technicians) an administrative personnel, responsible for the administration and operational control of the institutions. In that case personnel, in general, is employed and salaried by the institutions, even if they, like many of them do, maintain a certain professional autonomy. Some health care professionals work as free entrepreneurs in their own individual practices or in group practices. They receive their remuneration directly from their patients or from social security organizations. This mainly applies to physicians and certain paramedical professionals. In these practices, like in institutions, medical and other personnel can be employed in salaried positions. The **place of work** is an important parameter in studying health care manpower, because this provides at the same time indications of the services rendered and the structure of health care expenditure by type of activity (hospital care, ambulatory care).

Working hours

The production capacity of personnel not only depends on their numbers, but also on the time they devote to their professional activity. Not seldom statistics distinguish between full-time personnel and part-time personnel (but without indication of the precise duration of their activities) and combine these two categories in order to produce an evaluation of the size of personnel in terms of full-time equivalents.

Stock and flow

Personnel size varies in function of job entrances and exits. In every profession the number of job entrances is related to the number of certifications in previous years and, by consequence, to the number of students, admitted to corresponding studies. The number of job exits is related to the age structure and particularly to the proportion of persons of 60 years and older. Within the framework of prospective research concerning production capacity it is useful to know the numbers of students in different stages of their training and the **age structure** of active professionals.

Measuring activity

It has been stated already, that the measurement of numbers of personnel in terms of full-time equivalents is an approach of the production capacity of the different categories of personnel. Their activities, insofar as suitable, can be indicated by other parameters. This particularly applies to independent physicians and paramedical profesionnals, of whom it is possible to indicate the numbers of activities, classified in more or less detail in accordance with nomenclatures, existing at national level. In this field, considering the variablity of practices, it is difficult to find a unique, internationally comparable measure. Two examples:

pharmacists provide a more or less wide variety of products, deliver these products in different forms, prepacked or not and with different contents.

sometimes services of physicians can be calculated routinely according to a payment system per activity, but in other cases this information only is available from surveys or specific research. The meeting of physician and patient (doctors' session) seems to be the best unit for international comparisons. But it is necessary to realize, that such sessions have different durations per country and that they can consist of one or more examinations and connected treatments (injections, electrocardiograms, urine analysis).

Remuneration

In different countries personnel is remunerated according to different methods. These methods even can differ within countries for the same qualification, depending on the place of professional practice. Health care professionals generally are paid a salary or they receive fees per activity or per head. Methods of remuneration are based on a measure of the activity (time, treatment, category of patient) and on scales. International comparison can be based on unitary remunerations (doctors' session, a pharmaceutical product, one hour nursing), or on a total annual remuneration, crude or with professional costs deducted.

International comparison

For the purpose of international comparison statistics in general have to be based on rates, which can eliminate the role of exogenous factors, characteristic for every country (population, wealth, currency). In the case of manpower statistics parameters, permitting international comparison, are the densities in relation to the population (for example number of physicians per 1,000 inhabitants) or the specifications, expressed as a percentage of the total (for example proportion of general practitioners among all physicians). In case of monetary evaluation international comparison must have the ability to relate one currency with another (annual exchange rate or purchasing power parities) in order to transcribe remunerations in national currencies in one unique unit (for example ECU).

Establishment of comparative tables

The pioneer work done by OECD in the field of collection and harmonisation of statistics, which describe the health care systems of the member states, must be highly esteemed. The tables, published by this organization, constitute an important step, which already today proofs to be useful for governments in the appreciation of their systems of care.

There only will be amelioration and progress in the field of comparability of data, if every country directs his efforts in this sense.

For higher reasons, comparability of international statistics only can be assured, if tables with national data are based on figures, underlying identical definitions. This only can result from preceding international consultation and the start of particular efforts at national level in order to fulfil the need of the establishment of corresponding statistics. Today comparablity is assured for just a few parameters. In order to overcome this situation it is necessary to define nomenclatures, acceptable in the distinguished countries, which might create bridges between their national statistics and the harmonized statistics.

Below a list of tables is proposed, defined in two dimensions and with the unit indicated as discussed. These tables describe manpower, the remuneration of health care professionals. Also some examples of nomenclatures are presented, which correspond with different dimensions of the tables.

As a first step these tables could be submitted to the different countries in order to be filled in as good as possible, perhaps after adaptation in accordance with the national situation, confronting them with their own nomenclatures according to the previously indicated criteria (qualifications, place of work, demographic structures, activities).

In any case the tables shoud be returned, accompanied by notes, in which definitions and units used are described precisely and in which is explained, why tables have not been filled in and proposals for modifications are formulated.

All the answers should be analysed in order to reach a sub collection of uniform tables (and new tables, if needed), which might favour international comparison.

Note

[1)] Paper prepared for the first consultation "International comparison of Health Care Data", organized by CBS, Voorburg, 21–23 September 1994.

Proposal for a list of tables

Manpower tables

Table 1 Density of personnel by qualification
Unit: number per 1,000 inhabitants

Table 2 Number of students by attended study and progress in study
Unit: number per 1,000 inhabitants

Table 3 Age structure per qualification (3 age classes)
Unit: percentage; 100= total of the same qualification

Table 4 Division of manpower by place of work and by qualification
Unit: 100=total of a qualification

Tables of activity and remuneration

Table 5 Activity per person measured with different units, by qualification

Table 6 Sum of net remuneration before taxes per person, by qualification
Unit: ECU

Examples of nomenclatures: to be completed or to be simplified

Qualifications:

- Physicians, if possible by specialism
- Dentists
- Pharmacists
- Midwives
- Other health care personnel
  - Nurses (by specialty)
  - Physiotherapists
  - Therapists (speech, vision,..)
- Technical personnel
  - Engineers
  - Technicians
- Social personnel
- Administrative personnel

Nature of studies

Schools, training for different qualifications: medicine, pharmacy, dentistry, nursing.

Place of work

- Health care institutions with intramural care: hospitals of different categories (general, psychiatric, hospitals with other specialisms, institutions for the elderly.)
- Health centres for ambulatory care
- Independent professional practices
- Retail trade of medical goods

Activities

- Care
- Research, training
- Administration

Measurement of care activities

- number of services rendered
- number of patients
- working hours per day, week, year

Remuneration

Crude remuneration per unit (per service or other unit)
Net annual remuneration before taxes

Inputs and throughputs in in-patient care

by Jean-Pierre Poullier
OECD, Paris

1. Even within a "homogeneous" European Union grouping, comparisons of in-patient care pose formidable statistical problems. These relate foremost to boundaries, an issue dealt with under another heading of this workshop. Differences between Denmark (which has a relatively "narrow" list of *institutions* classified as providing medical and paramedical benefits) and the Netherlands (which has an "extensive" list of *institutions* classified as providing somatic and mental benefits) may explain close to half of the two percentage points differences in GDP shares between this pair of countries. Boundaries are not the only issue.

2. The area is fraught with conceptual, definitional and measurement issues. A few are alluded to below, using as quantitative exhibits data on "acute" care. This is in order to by-pass part of the boundary issue. "Acute" is, however, not a homogeneous concept among the six countries considered in this workshop.

3. Hospitals appear to have never been defined: they are institutions which granted themselves that label or which were granted this label by a Ministry of Health or by a statistical agency. Beds have not been defined either, nor have important measurement criteria such as "what is an appropriate estimate of the stock of beds?", "how should bed occupancy be measured?". Definitional issues will first be examined before a few trends and comparative issues are studied.

4. No internationally agreed-on definition of "acute care" exists. To get the ball rolling, the OECD Secretariat proposed "hospitals with a length of stay below 28 days or with actual stay below 28 days". This measure had some relevance in the 1950s. It is of limited value in the 1990s. The bulk of somatic care and of mental disturbances treated in OECD countries "general" hospitals refer to patients hospitalised for less than two weeks. The average spreads between 5.2 days in the country with the recorded lowest average stay (Australia) among the 25 OECD countries and 13.4 in the countries with the recorded highest mean stay (Germany and Switzerland). For the six countries concerned by this exercise, the current record (source: OECD Health Systems: Facts and Trends, Paris, 1993) is presented in table 1.

The German observations refer to the pre-reunification territory of the Federal Republic. Since 1990, a new classification applies in Germany in which the concept of acute care no longer constitutes a standard disaggregation.

Table 1 ALOS (in days)

	1985	1990
Belgium	10.9*	8.7
Denmark	7.8	6.6
France	8.3	7.7
Germany	13.9	13.4
Netherlands	12.5	11.2
Switzerland	14.7	13.4

* 1986.

5. As much as possible, the estimates are "mid-year", i.e. beds at 1st January of two consecutive years added up and divided by two in order to represent an annual average. The population denominator is an annual average when the figure is calculated by the OECD Secretariat. Many (most?) hospitals in industrialised countries compile their capacity on a daily basis: beds available for patient care. None of the six countries in this exercise indicates that its reported bed stock is calculated as an average daily census. For comparisons (as well as for domestic reporting purposes), would average daily census not be a preferable concept?

6. As is evident from the first exhibit, the "28 day" concept is no longer a discriminating concept. Denmark proposed to substitute a concept based on the number of services performed by hospital-based physicians. The rationale is that in "acute care" institutions contacts with patients are frequent, while in "chronic care" institutions it is a much smaller number. There are, however, no readily available data in the other five countries to add to the Danish-Norwegian comparison reported in OECD Health Systems: Facts and Trends, Chapter 4. A practical proposal for this exercise would be for the Danish participants to this exercise to put on the table a worksheet of the kind used for the Denmark-Norway comparison and to ask the other five participants to fill it as much as possible if a meaningful discussion on a potential alternative were to be estimated quickly.

Table 2 Admission rate

	(% of population)		Staff per bed		Nurses per bed	
	1985	1990	1985	1990	1985	1990
Belgium	15.3	16.8	1.10	1.46*	0.63	0.82*
Denmark	19.2	20.6	2.30	2.83	0.60	0.81
France	18.9	20.7	0.98	1.09	0.35	0.38**
Germany	17.4	18.5	1.21	1.31**	0.42	0.48**
Netherlands	10.9	10.3	1.93	2.13	0.82	0.87**
Switzerland	13.5	13.9	1.78	1.91	0.95	0.98

** 1991.
** 1989.

7. The reference to physician-patient contacts brings to the fore the fact that the health legislation as well as actual medical practice differ sensibly across (and within) countries. This is shown for three variables in table 2 on page 287.

8. Admissions are not number of people entering into a hospital in the given year but the number of episodes divided by the population. Episodes refer in theory to continuous periods of stay plus readmissions for the same episode within a two-week period following the previous discharge. Is this practice adhered to in the real world? Are differences in admissions not also reflecting the wider diffusion of diagnostic equipment in some countries (i.e. ambulatory procedures) than in others? How are ambulatory surgery, day cases, minimally invasive therapies, treated: admission for less than a day or exclusion from hospital statistics? Data on the prevalence of these approaches are desirable; they are not at this time.

9. In some countries, external contracting for ancillary and catering services is a frequent occurrence; in others, it is a more recent phenomenon. In some countries, hospitals have sizeable ambulance fleets; in others, these services are contracted. Union lines of demarcation require in some countries the recruitment of a large number of auxiliaries; in others, hospital workers may exert a larger number of functions. Nurses vary in the range of responsibilities they are allowed to carry out. Could each one of these be succinctly described in individual country notes?

10. The prevalence of full-time employment differs between the six countries as do definitions of full-time employment equivalents. Actual definition are not spelled out: conventional working hours range, it seems, from 35 to 44 hours, part-time employment from 12 to 27 hours weekly, but conventions regarding night and week-end shifts vary. Could these be spelled out and be transparent?

11. What are the prevailing categories of employment in each country? Are nurses defined as persons with at least two years of post-secondary school education, at the exclusion of helpers and of dedicated but untrained staff? Are midwives included under nurses? Are staff and nurses a count of persons or full-time equivalents? How are part-timers aggregated into full-time staff? What is the degree of subcontracting?

12. The use of hospital equipment varies considerably (see table 3 on page289). Part of these differences noted relate to the heterogeneity of the underlying bed concepts. "Acute care" means not only different case-mix concepts across the six countries. It relates in part to cultural mores and economic incentives with respect to early discharges. Variations in common medical care practice are sizeable within and across countries, as shown by data for average length of stay and for discharge rates by ICD (International Classification of Disease) classes. Similar data are available for detailed codes at the three digit ICD level, but the message is similar (only a sample of codes is shown in table 4 to 7).

Table 3 Use of hospital equipment

	Turnover per bed (episodes of care per bed)		Occupancy rate (%)	
	1985	1990	1985	1990
Belgium	18.2	23.3	83.3*	81.9
Denmark	35.6	42.6	81.6	81.6
France	27.1	31.4**	77.9	77.3
Germany	18.0	20.0**	85.0	86.4
Netherlands	23.0	23.8	79.1	73.3
Switzerland	19.8	21.5	80.0	79.0

** 1986. ** 1989.

Table 4 Average length of stay by ICD-chapters, 1985 (France 1986)

		Bel	Den	Fra	Ger	Net	Swi
Infectious and parasatic diseases	(001–139)	..	7.3	9.3	17.9	14.7	13.0
Neoplasms	(140–239)	..	9.0	10.4	16.2	15.6	16.7
Endocrine and metabolic diseases	(240–279)	..	10.0	9.9	20.3	17.0	20.4
Diseases of the blood	(280–289)	..	8.8	8.1	16.3	13.0	12.1
Mental disorders	(290–319)	..	11.2	10.3	35.6	35.1	20.0
Diseases of the nervous system	(320–389)	..	7.9	7.8	16.0	10.3	14.7
Diseases of the circulatory system	(390–459)	..	13.2	11.3	21.1	14.6	19.7
Diseases of the respiratory system	(460–519)	..	7.8	7.1	13.2	10.1	13.1
Diseases of the digestive system	(520–579)	..	7.2	8.0	15.5	12.6	12.1
Diseases of the genito-urinary system	(580–629)	..	5.9	6.5	13.2	9.2	9.6
Complications of pregnancy and childbirth	(630–676)	..	4.8	7.0	7.4	7.0	7.8
Diseases of the skin and subcutaneous tissue	(680–709)	..	8.7	8.2	18.5	15.9	13.3
Diseases of the musculo-skeletal system	(710–739)	..	12.0	9.3	21.4	12.2	16.5
Congenital anomalies	(740–759)	..	6.0	7.7	14.3	9.4	10.8
Certain causes of perinatal morbidity	(760–779)	..	10.7	15.4	20.4	11.2	13.2
Symptoms of ill-defined conditions	(780–799)	..	6.4	6.8	15.7	10.5	8.8
Accidents, poisoning and violence	(800–999)	..	8.7	7.5	16.2	14.7	13.5
All other		..	4.2	5.2	..	6.3	8.2
All categories	(001–999)	..	8.1	8.3	17.0	12.0	14.5

Table 5 Average length of stay by ICD-chapters, 1990 (Belgium 1988)

		Bel	Den	Fra	Ger	Net	Swi
Infectious and parasatic diseases	(001–139)	9.0	6.3	..	..	13.2	11.6
Neoplasms	(140–239)	11.6	7.5	..	..	13.5	15.0
Endocrine and metabolic diseases	(240–279)	11.0	9.0	..	..	14.5	20.2
Diseases of the blood	(280–289)	9.4	6.8	..	..	11.2	12.5
Mental disorders	(290–319)	16.8	9.7	..	..	34.8	19.7
Diseases of the nervous system	(320–389)	8.2	6.1	..	..	8.2	13.3
Diseases of the circulatory system	(390–459)	11.3	10.6	..	..	12.9	17.4
Diseases of the respiratory system	(460–519)	8.4	6.6	..	..	9.9	12.5
Diseases of the digestive system	(520–579)	8.4	5.9	..	..	10.9	10.8
Diseases of the genito-urinary system	(580–629)	6.8	4.7	..	..	8.5	8.8
Complications of pregnancy and childbirth	(630–676)	6.8	3.8	..	..	6.0	7.4
Diseases of the skin and subcutaneous tissue	(680–709)	12.2	7.9	..	..	14.4	13.0
Diseases of the musculo-skeletal system	(710–739)	9.9	10.1	..	..	10.1	15.4
Congenital anomalies	(740–759)	7.2	5.2	..	..	8.8	10.0
Certain causes of perinatal morbidity	(760–779)	12.4	9.6	..	..	9.6	11.9
Symptoms of ill-defined conditions	(780–799)	6.3	5.3	..	..	9.2	9.2
Accidents, poisoning and violence	(800–999)	9.2	7.9	..	..	13.6	12.2
All other		6.2	3.6	..	..	5.7	..
All categories	(001–999)	9.3	6.7	..	..	..	13.3

Table 6 Discharge rates by ICD-chapters, 1985

		Bel	Den	Fra	Ger	Net	Swi
Infectious and parasatic diseases	(001–139)	..	..	..	..	..	..
Neoplasms	(140–239)	..	..	..	..	9.1	..
Endocrine and metabolic diseases	(240–279)	..	..	..	..	..	..
Diseases of the blood	(280–289)	..	..	..	..	..	..
Mental disorders	(290–319)	..	..	..	..	..	..
Diseases of the nervous system	(320–389)	..	..	..	..	..	..
Diseases of the circulatory system	(390–459)	..	..	..	..	13.5	..
Diseases of the respiratory system	(460–519)	..	..	..	..	7.6	..
Diseases of the digestive system	(520–579)	..	..	..	..	9.5	..
Diseases of the genito-urinary system	(580–629)	..	..	..	..	3.2	..
Complications of pregnancy and childbirth	(630–676)	..	..	..	..	17.2	..
Diseases of the skin and subcutaneous tissue	(680–709)	..	..	..	..	..	..
Diseases of the musculo-skeletal system	(710–739)	..	..	..	..	..	..
Congenital anomalies	(740–759)	..	..	..	..	..	..
Certain causes of perinatal morbidity	(760–779)	..	..	..	..	..	..
Symptoms of ill-defined conditions	(780–799)	..	..	..	..	..	..
Accidents, poisoning and violence	(800–999)	..	..	..	..	7.9	..
All other		..	..	..	..	..	..
All categories	(001–999)	..	..	..	..	..	..

Table 7 Discharge rates by ICD-chapters, 1990

		Bel	Den	Fra	Ger	Net	Swi
Infectious and parasatic diseases	(001–139)	..	..	..	..	1.1	..
Neoplasms	(140–239)	..	..	..	..	9.3	..
Endocrine and metabolic diseases	(240–279)	..	..	..	..	2.2	..
Diseases of the blood	(280–289)	..	..	..	..	0.9	..
Mental disorders	(290–319)	..	..	..	..	1.5	..
Diseases of the nervous system	(320–389)	..	..	..	..	5.9	..
Diseases of the circulatory system	(390–459)	..	..	..	..	14.2	..
Diseases of the respiratory system	(460–519)	..	..	..	..	6.9	..
Diseases of the digestive system	(520–579)	..	..	..	..	8.5	..
Diseases of the genito-urinary system	(580–629)	..	..	..	..	6.8	..
Complications of pregnancy and childbirth	(630–676)	..	..	..	..	16.8	..
Diseases of the skin and subcutaneous tissue	(680–709)	..	..	..	..	1.3	..
Diseases of the musculo-skeletal system	(710–739)	..	..	..	..	9.9	..
Congenital anomalies	(740–759)	..	..	..	..	1.3	..
Certain causes of perinatal morbidity	(760–779)	..	..	..	..	3.5	..
Symptoms of ill-defined conditions	(780–799)	..	..	..	..	5.6	..
Accidents, poisoning and violence	(800–999)	..	..	..	..	7.3	..
All other		..	..	..	..	3.4	..
All categories	(001–999)	..	..	..	..	152.7	..

Table 8 Mean length of stay by ICD disease categories, 1985 (France 1986)

		Bel	Den	Fra	Ger	Net	Swi
Pulmonary tuberculosis	(011)	..	20.6	23.3	64.3	33.6	36.6
Trachea, bronchus and lung cancer	(162)	..	11.7	11.5	18.2	17.1	16.2
Breast cancer	(174)	..	8.7	9.5	13.5	16.6	18.7
Prostate cancer	(185)	..	12.5	13.5	19.9	16.1	19.3
Diabetes mellitus	(250)	..	10.9	11.4	25.1	18.5	25.5
Cataract	(366)	..	5.7	7.2	..	..	11.1
Otitis	(380–382)	..	5.3	7.1	13.1	8.6	12
Hypertension	(401–405)	..	9.4	13	..	14.4	16.2
Acute myocardial infarction	(410)	..	9.1	10.3	21.9	14.1	15.8
Pneumonia	(480–486)	..	10.7	11.7	21.5	14.8	17.3
Bronchitis	(490–491)	..	11.7	..	20.3	17.4	17.1
Asthma	(483)	..	11.6	11.2	20.2	18.3	19.6
Ulcers of stomach & small intestine	(531–534)	..	6.8	8.3	20.2	13.3	15.1
Appendicitis	(540–543)	..	7.3	10.2	20.4	18.1	14.1
Inguinal hernia	(550–554)	..	4.7	7.1	10.3	9.2	9.1
Cholelithiasis	(574)	..	..	8.7	14.2	8.3	..
Nephritis	(580–584)	..	10.9	11.5	20	16.1	14.2
Calculus of kidney and ureter	(592)	..	9.7	6.3	21.1	20.2	16.3
Cystitis	(595)	..	6.7	5.9	12.6	10.2	7.4
Normal delivery	(650)	..	7.5	5.7	15.2	10.4	11.6
Major puerperal infection	(670)	..	4.7	7.1	7.3	4.7	8.5

Table 9 Mean length of stay by ICD disease categories, 1990 (Belgium 1988)

		Bel	Den	Fra	Ger	Net	Swi
Pulmonary tuberculosis	(011)	19.1	13.1	..	..	..	25.7
Trachea, bronchus and lung cancer	(162)	11.2	..	..	..	14.6	14.9
Breast cancer	(174)	11.7	7.2	..	..	12.9	17.2
Prostate cancer	(185)	13.8	10.4	..	..	13.3	15.9
Diabetes mellitus	(250)	11.9	10.5	..	..	16.2	24.3
Cataract	(366)	..	4.0	..	..	..	13.3
Otitis	(380–382)	6.5	3.2	..	..	5.0	7.2
Hypertension	(401–405)	12.1	9.0	..	..	..	..
Acute myocardial infarction	(410)	9.5	7.8	..	..	..	..
Pneumonia	(480–486)	12.5	8.0	..	..	12.7	15.1
Bronchitis	(490–491)	11.8	8.9	..	..	16.1	15.6
Asthma	(483)	13.0	10.4	..	..	17.1	..
Ulcers of stomach & small intestine	(531–534)	8.6	6.0	..	..	11.3	14.9
Appendicitis	(540–543)	11.4	6.1	..	..	..	..
Inguinal hernia	(550–554)	6.6	4.3	..	..	7.8	8.0
Cholelithiasis	(574)	7.7	3.7	..	..	..	..
Nephritis	(580–584)	12.6	8.0	..	..	12.2	12.8
Calculus of kidney and ureter	(592)	10.1	9.8	..	..	..	..
Cystitis	(595)	5.5	4.4	..	..	6.6	6.6
Normal delivery	(650)	7.9	6.8	..	..	8.6	12.0
Major puerperal infection	(670)	7.0	3.8	..	..	3.7	7.6

13. Length of stay, even accounting for statistical vagaries, vary considerably (see table 8 and 9 on page 291). The Danish and Dutch data are a national sample. The French is an experimental national sample. The German data relate to AOK or local sickness funds, possibly a higher level than that for the total GKV (sickness insurance funds) universe since it may include an older than average or a sicker than average segment of the total population. The Swiss data originate from the Hospital Federation Statistics, deemed to comprise a little over 85 % of all episodes of care. The Belgian 1988 entries are an experimental national sample. A 1:2 (or higher) ratio is found for all ICD classes. Variations reach 1:3 (or more) at a finer (three digit) levels (e.g. pulmonary tuberculosis), 1:2 (e.g. diabetis), and so on.

14. Discharge rates are being collated for the same ICD chapters and ICD subcategories. They exhibit large variations, too. At this stage, for the six countries of this study, data have been accessed only for the Netherlands. (Since discharge rates are readily accessible for the other five countries, the workshop participants are invited to fill the column of their country of origin and supply a copy to Netherlands Statistics in order to fill the table and distribute it as a room document.)

15. Once differences in ALOS and in discharge rates have been ascertained as "statistically" homogeneous, the next step in the comparison requires reasonably homogeneous cost data. Only a very crude approximation can be obtained from aggregate acute care expenditure converted at purchasing power parity (for this exercise, an aggregate PPP was used, as reliable medical specific PPP are still some way off – see OECD Health Systems: Facts and Trends, volume 2, annex 2). Few among the six countries readily supply the required data.

Table 10 Acute hospital care expenditure 1985 and 1990: alternative concepts in $PPP

	Per inhabitant		Per bed ($)		Per day ($)	
	1985	1990	1985	1990	1985	1990
Belgium	. .	. .	. .	. .	. .	. .
Denmark	374	437*	74,255	93,180*	. .	. .
France	503	670	88,869	129,877	76	104
Germany	. .	. .	. .	. .		
Netherlands	309	413	65,498	95,618	. .	
Switzerland**	353	585	52,141	90,648	143	248

** 1989.
** 1984 (different source from 1990 base estimate).

16. As for ALOS and discharge rates, dispersions are considerable. Disaggregation by ICD chapters or codes are difficult. None of the six countries appears to be calculating these at ICD class level. Five of the six countries appear, however, to be experimenting with case-mix measures (Diagnosis Related Groups,

Groupes Homognes de maladies, Patient Mix Classification, Health Related Groups). These may shed some light on the dispersion. To the extent possible, participants to the workshop are invited to supply data, for a recent year, on discharge rates, on length of stay and on costs for a range of diagnoses corresponding as closely as possible to the sample proposed in the attached tables on ALOS.

Table 11 Mean length of stay by case-mix (Diagnosis-Related Groups), 1988, in days

		Bel	Den	Fra	Ger	Net	Swi
Diagnosis-related groups (DRG-codes)							
Specific cerebrovascular disorders	(14)	21.3	..	15.8	..	..	..
Lens procedures	(39)	6.4	..	8.2	..	..	..
Extra-ocular procedures, except orbit	(41)	2.7	..	3.0	..	..	..
Miscellaneous ear, nose andthroat procedures	(55)	4.3	..	6.9	..	..	..
Tonsillectomy and/or adenoidectomy	(60)	1.9	..	1.8	..	..	..
Otitis media	(70)	4.9	..	3.5	..	..	..
Respiratory neoplasms	(82)	10.4	..	10.6	..	..	..
Chronic obstructive pulmonary disorders	(88)	14.3	..	11.3	..	..	..
Bronchitis and asthma	(98)	7.0	..	3.8	..	..	..
Circulatory disorders with acute infarction	(122)	10.8	..	12.7	..	..	..
Heart failure and shock	(127)	15.2	..	14.1	..	..	..
Angina pectoris	(140)	9.1	..	9.6	..	..	..
Inguinal and femoral hernia procedures	(162)	7.7	..	8.1	..	..	..
Appendicectomy	(167)	6.1	..	9.6	..	..	..
Esophagitis, gastroenteritis, age 70+	(182)	10.4	..	10.5	..	..	..
Knee procedures	(222)	13.3	..	8.9	..	..	..
Foot procedures	(225)	4.2	..	9.3	..	..	..
Hand procedures except ganglions	(229)	6.9	..	6.3	..	..	..
Medical back problems	(243)	3.3	..	7.6	..	..	..
Diabetis, age 36+	(294)	7.3	..	5.4	..	..	..
Non-radical hysterectomy	(355)	11.2	..	6.7	..	..	..
Caesarean section	(371)	12.3	..	2.6	..	..	..
Vaginal delivery without complications	(373)	7.0	..	..	..	..	..
Normal newborns	(391)	2.7	..	..	..	..	..

The information would be needed for separations (discharges) as % of relevant population, for ALOS (as above) and for cost per discharge.

17. Many instant comparisons provide "definitive" explanations on costs and output in the health industries of adjacent countries. The examples shown indicate that, at this stage, only crude approximations can be supplied. More attention will have to be given to definitions and cultural variables, such as those shown above. These are offered as a sample to be enriched during the discussions and as an incentive to make more details available, when producing numbers.

Data on the supply of health care

C.J.P.M. van Mosseveld
J.M. Smit

Introduction

This paper is written in view of the first consultation of the project "International comparability of health care data" in September 1994. It deals with the supply of health care provisions.

Data on health care are in the middle of interest. Without any doubt you will be familiar with stories in papers on increasing cost and cost-containment in the field of health care. These issues are at the top of the political agenda because of the burden of health expenditure on national budgets. The share of total health expenditure in total domestic expenditure in 1991 varies for the OECD-countries between 4.1% in Turkey and 13.9% in the United States. The health-to-total expenditure ratio concentrates in the 7 to 8% range. A closer look at the six participating countries shows that the health-to-total expenditure ratio varies between 6.7% in Denmark and 9.4% in Germany.

Looking at these figures we must of course be aware of the difficulties at comparing international data. Differences in boundaries, concepts, definitions, estimating methodologies and nomenclatures make it hard to compare the data of different countries. Comparisons over time and across countries are powerful means of examining each national health system. So the above mentioned problems have to be overcome by finding solutions for these differences. This paper concentrates on indicators concerning the supply of health care.

Methodology

Supply is only relevant in connection with demand. In the service sector (like the health care sector) stock production is not possible. The (explicit) demand for services results in most cases directly in supply for services. Of course it is possible on the one hand that the total supply (capacity of production) is not used to its fullest; on the other hand total demand can exceed total supply (resulting in waiting lists).

In a system of (integrated) health statistics the statistics on the problem (health and sickness on the population level leading to demand), the health care provisions (supply) and the demanded respectively supplied services are coherently presented.

In this paper supply is directly linked to the capacity of institutions, the number of employees in institutions and the number of independent health care professionals in the field of health care. For comparability reasons generally accepted denominators are needed. Keeping this in mind an attempt is made to construct a set of variables regarding supply that is suitable for international comparison. The number of variables concerning supply is rather limited. As sources the OECD Health System and the list of variables of the Ministry of Health, Welfare and Sports is used, supplemented by some data on supply in the Dutch publication on Cost and Financing of Health Care. The objective of our working-method is to locate remarkable differences between the participating countries, in order to become aware of differences in health care systems (e.g. concepts of health care, health care organisation).

Although in this paper data on extramural health care are presented, the main objective of this paper is to feed the discussion on the comparison of intramural health care.

Set of variables

The chosen variables on supply can be grouped in an intramural (semimural included) and an extramural block.

For the provisions in the intramural health care we used the number of beds per thousand of the population. For the extramural health care we have used the number of independent professionals for some categories of care.

In addition to these international available data figures are presented concerning the number of persons employed (in full time equivalents) per bed in some categories of intramural health care in the Netherlands.

Results

To give some insight at macro level table 1 supplies data on the total employment in health care per thousand of the population for the six countries participating in this project. The ratio in the six countries (as far as available) varies from 18.0 in Belgium to 42.8 in Switzerland in 1985.

In table 2 the number of beds per thousand of the population are presented for some categories of intramural health care in the six countries. Striking are the differences between the six countries especially in the categories general hospitals (short stay hospitals) and nursing homes.

For general hospitals the share of beds per thousand of the population varies from 4.7 (Netherlands) to 6.7 (Germany) in 1985. The same differences can be seen in 1990. For nursing homes the share ranges from 1.2 (France) to 3.5 (Netherlands) in 1990.

Furthermore in the comparison of the years 1985 and 1990 there are considerable changes in these shares in some countries. In Belgium e.g. a substitution between hospital beds and nursing home beds seems likely.

In table 3 the number of independent health care professionals per thousand of the population for some categories of extramural health care in the six countries are presented. The differences in the share of physicians per thousand of population can probably be explained by the corresponding differences in the share of general practitioners per thousand of the population. A wide range is also present in the number of pharmacists per thousand of the population. In the period 1985 - 1990 no great changes in the relative differences can be recorded.

A probable explanation for the differences could be that the activities (functions) and the position of general practitioners and pharmacists in health care are different in the countries.

For the Netherlands an additional variable is mentioned in table 4. This variable concerns the number of persons employed (in full time equivalents) per bed in some categories of intramural health care. This variable gives some insight in the intensity of the provided care.

Concluding remarks

The number of available variables for international comparison on the supply of intramural health care is very limited. The presented variables give some insight in the possible differences in the definition and organisation of health care between the six countries. This information on itself is not enough to draw conclusions. The information must be used in combination with the information in the activity-matrices and the country-profiles to be able to make progress in international comparability of health care data.

Table 1
Total employment in health care per 1,000 of the population

	1985	1990
Netherlands	21.1	22.2
Belgium	18.0	
France [1]	26.0	
Germany	18.2	20.8
Denmark	20.6	21.2
Switzerland	42.3	

[1] France data for 1986 instead of 1985.

Table 2
Number of beds in intramural health care per 1,000 of the population

	General hospitals		Psychiatric hospitals		Nursing homes	
	1985	1990	1985	1990	1985	1990
Netherlands	4.7	4.3	1.7	1.6	3.4	3.5
Belgium [1]	5.8	4.9	2.1	1.9	0.5	1.2
France	5.7	5.2	2.0	1.7	1.0	1.2
Germany	5.9	6.0	1.8	1.4	1.7	2.8
Denmark	5.0	4.6	1.5	0.7		
Switzerland	6.7	6.5	2.0	1.5		

[1] Belgium nursing homes 1986 instead of 1985.

Table 3
Number of health care professionals per 1,000 of the population

	Physicians		General practitioners		Dentists		Pharmacists	
	1985	1990	1985	1990	1985	1990	1985	1990
Netherlands	2.2	2.5	0.4	0.4	0.5	0.5	0.1	0.2
Belgium	2.8	3.2	1.4	1.5	0.6	0.7	1.1	1.2
France	2.2	2.6	1.3	1.4	0.6	0.7	0.8	0.9
Germany	2.6	2.5	0.9	0.9	0.5	0.5	0.4	0.5
Denmark	2.5	2.8	0.6	0.6	0.5	0.5	0.2	0.2
Switzerland [1]	2.7	2.9	0.5	0.6	0.4	0.4		0.5

[1] Switzerland GP 1986 instead of 1985.

Table 4
Additional key variables for the Netherlands

	Persons employed (in FTE) per bed	
	1985	1990
Intramural sector		
Hospitals	1.9	2.1
Psychiatric hospitals	1.1	1.2
Mentally deficients	0.9	1.0
Nursing Homes	1.1	1.1

Literature

1. Adams et al., "De eigen bijdrage in de gezondheidszorg in de Europese gemeenschap", Antwerpen-Apeldoorn, 1992
2. Adams, M., "Ziekenfonds over de grens", Antwerpen-Apeldoorn, 1992
3. BIGE, "Compendium Gezondheidsstatistiek 1992", Brussel, 1992
4. BIGE, "Compendium Gezondheidsstatistiek 1994", Brussel, 1994
5. Bocognano, A. and Raffy-Pihan, N., "L'emploi dans le secteur de la santé; évolution 1982–1992", CREDES, Paris, 1995
6. Boerma, W.G.W., de Jong, F.A.J.M., Mulder, P.H., Health care and general practice across Europe, NIVEL, Utrecht, 1993
7. Boot, J.M., Knapen, M.H.J.M., "De Nederlandse Gezondheidszorg", Utrecht, 1993.
8. Centraal Bureau voor de Statistiek, "Vademecum Gezondheidsstatistiek Nederland 1996", Voorburg / Heerlen, 1996 (yearly publication)
9. Centraal Bureau voor de Statistiek / Statistics Netherlands, "Kosten en financiering van de gezondheidszorg 1996" / "Cost and Financing of health care 1996", Voorburg / Heerlen, 1997 (yearly publication)
10. Centraal Bureau voor de Statistiek / Statistics Netherlands, "Intramurale Gezondheidszorg 1996" / "Intramural Health care 1993", Voorburg / Heerlen, 1997 (yearly publication)
11. Davidse, W, Wissink, G.J., "Functioneren artsenlaboratoria in Nederland", Leiden, 1986
12. Delnoij, D.M.J. et al., "Brancherapport curatieve somatische zorg", NIVEL/NZI, Utrecht, 1996
13. Delnoij, Diana M.J., "Home care in Germany" in "Home care in Europe", edited by Hutten, J.B.F. and Kerkstra, A., p. 130–149, Aldershot, 1996.
14. Deramon, Jean, Volovitch, Pierre, "Systèmes de Santé; une comparaison Allemagne, France, Royaume-Uni; chiffres repères", Ministère des Affaires Sociales, de la Santé, et de la Ville, Paris, 1993
15. Duriez, M., Sandier, S., "Le système de Santé, en France; Organisation et Fonctionnement", Paris, 1994
16. Service des Statistiques, des Etudes et des Systèmes d'Information, "Comptes Nationaux de la Santé, 1990–1991–1992", Ministère des Affaires Sociales, de la Santé, et de la Ville, Paris, 1993
17. Escoyez P., Met argusogen. Ingreep in thuiszorg een precedent?, Artsenkrant, vol. 17, nr. 984, p.5.
18. Financieel Overzicht Zorg 1996, Den Haag, 1995 (and earlier editions)
19. Ham, P.J. v.d., "Transmurale zorg en artsenlaboratoria", Medisch Contact, jrg. 49, nr. 45, 11 november 1994

20. Hausser, D., Jeangros, C., Martin, J., "La consultation médicale", Genève: Médecine et Hygiène, 1990.
21. Hingstman, L. en Harmsen, J. , "Beroepen in de extramurale gezondheidszorg 1994", Utrecht, 1994.
22. Hoffmann, Dr. U., "Zum Aufbau einer nationalen Gesundheitsberichterstattung", Wirtschaft und Statistik, 1/1993, p. 33–42
23. Hutten, J.B.F., "Home care in Belgium" in "Home care in Europe", edited by Hutten, J.B.F. and Kerkstra, A., p. 62–81, Aldershot, 1996.
24. Jau, Jürg., "Mitglieder-Statistik 1993 der Verbindung der Schweizer Aerzte", Separatdruck. In: Schweizerische Aerztezeitung, Band 75, Heft 19.. Bern, Göttingen, Toronto, Seattle: Hans Huber, 1994: 756–773 / "Statistique 1993 des membres de la Fédération des médecins suisses". Tirage part. In: Bulletin des médecins suisses, 19. Berne, Göttingen, Toronto, Seattle: Hans Huber, 1994: 756–773
25. Kemenade, Y.W. van, "Health Care in Europe", Nationale Raad voor de Volksgezondheid, Zoetermeer, 1993
26. Kerkstra, K., "Home care in the Netherlands" in "Home care in Europe", edited by Hutten, J.B.F. and Kerkstra, A., p. 130–149, Aldershot, 1996.
27. Ministère des Affaires Sociales, de la Santé et de la Ville, Service des Statistiques, des Etudes et des Systèmes d'Information, "Comptes Nationaux de la Santé 1992-1993-1994", Paris, 1995 (yearly publication)
28. Ministère de la Santé Publique et de l'Environnement, "La santé dans la Belgique fédérale et ses communautés; situation actuelle et tendances", Bruxelles, 1993
29. Ministerie van Volksgezondheid en Leefmilieu, "Gezondheid in het federale België en zijn gemeenschappen", Brussel, 1993
30. Ministère de la Santé Publique et de l'Environnement, "Annuaire statistique des hôpitaux, situation au 1er janvier 1993, Bruxelles
31. Ministère de la Santé Publique et de l'Environnement, "Annuaire statistique des hôpitaux, origine des patients hospitalisés, exercice 1992", Bruxelles
32. Ministry of Health, "Health Care in Denmark", Copenhagen, 1993
33. Mosseveld, C.J.P.M. van, Son, P. van, "International comparison of health care data; Phase 1: Intramural health care", Statistics Netherlands, Voorburg / Heerlen, 1996
34. Mosseveld, C.J.P.M. van, Son, P. van, "Advanced Medico-Technological Procedures", Statistics Netherlands, Voorburg / Heerlen, 1997
35. Mosseveld, C.J.P.M. van, Son, P. van, "Transport of Patients", Statistics Netherlands, Voorburg / Heerlen, 1998.
36. Mosseveld, C.J.P.M. van, Son, P. van, "International comparison of health care data; Phase II: Extramural health care, prevention, medical goods and other services", Statistics Netherlands, Voorburg / Heerlen, 1998 (participants edition)
37. Müller, Dr.J., "Duitsland doet het gründlich", Inzet, april 1994, p. 17–19.

38. Müller, Stefan et al., "Zahlenspiegel der Sozialen Sicherheit der Schweiz", Ausgabe 1994. M+S.Bern: Bundesamt für Sozialversicherung, 1994
39. Nationale Raad voor de Volksgezondheid, Y.W. van Kemenade, "Health Care in Europe", Zoetermeer, 1993.
40. NIVEL, Boerma, W.G.W., de Jong, F.A.J.M., Mulder, P.H., Health care and general practice across Europe Utrecht, 1993
41. Nonneman, W., Doorslaer, E. van, "The role of the sickness funds in the Belgian health care market", Soc. Sci. Med., vol. 39, no 10, pp. 1483–1495.
42. OECD, Hurst, J.,"The Reform of Health Care; a comparative analysis of seven OECD countries", Paris, 1992
43. OECD, "Health systems, facts and trends 1960–1991", Paris, 1993
44. OECD, Health Data Bank, 1997 and previous versions, Paris, 1997
45. Rössel, Raymond, "Kosten des Gesundheitswesens. Ergebnisse 1985–1991 und Schätzung 1992-1995", Statistik der Schweiz, Gesundheit. Bern: Bundesamt für Statistik, 1994 / "Coûts du système de santé. Résultats 1985–1991 et estimation 1992-1995", Statistique de la Suisse, Santé. Berne: Office fédéral de la statistique, 1994.
46. Rössel Raymond, "Kosten des Gesundheitswesens. Entwicklung in der Periode 1960–1995 und aktuelle detaillierte Ergebnisse", Statistik der Schweiz, Gesundheit. Bern: Bundesamt für Statistik, 1996/"Coûts du système de santé. Evolution durant la période 1960 à 1995 et résultats détaillés récents", Statistique de la Suisse, Santé. Berne: Office fédéral de la statistique, 1996.
47. Sachverständigenrat für die Konzertierte Aktion in Gesundheitswesen, Jahresgutachten 1992, "Ausbau in Deutschland und Aufbruch nach Europa", Baden-Baden, 1992
48. Schneider et al., "Gesundheitssysteme im internationalen Vergleich", BASYS, Augsburg, 1993/1995
49. Schrijvers, A.J.P. (editor), "Health and Health Care in the Netherlands", Utrecht, 1997
50. Schweizerische Kommission für Gesundheitsstatistik, "Organisatorische Leitgedanken und Empfehlungen", Statistik der Schweiz, Gesundheit. Bern: Bundesamt für Statistik, 1994 / Commission Suisse de Statistiques Sanitaires. "Lignes directrices et recommandations", Statistique de la Suisse, Santé. Berne: Office fédéral de la statistique, 1994.
51. SFA (Schweiz. Fachstelle für Alkohol- und andere Drogenprobleme) SAMBAD, Ambulante Suchtberatung 1994, Lausanne: SFA, 1996.
52. Spinnewyn, H., Pacolet, J., "Financiële stromen en werkgelegenheid in de gezondheidszorg in Vlaanderen", Leuven, 1993
53. Swiss Institute for Public Health, "Highlights on Health in Switzerland", Lausanne: Swiss Institute for Public Health, 1993.
54. Verheij, R.A., "Home care in France" in "Home care in Europe", edited by Hutten, J.B.F. and Kerkstra, A., p. 116–129, Aldershot, 1996.

55. VESKA, "Das schweizerische Krankenhauswesen im Spiegel der Statistik 1991", In: Schweizer Spital, 11. Aarau, 1992 (56 p.).
56. VESKA-Statistikzentrale, Veska Panorama, "Das schweizerische Krankenhauswesen 1991 in Zahlen. Kommentar, Tabellen und Grafiken", Aarau: Veska, 1993 (24 p.).
57. Voorlichtingscentrum Sociale Verzekering, "De kleine gids voor de Nederlandse sociale zekerheid 1994", Deventer, 1994
58. Vreugdenhil, Drs. J.C., Bruine, Drs. M. de, "Gezondheidszorg in Europa", Rotterdam, 1992
59. Werff, Prof. Dr. A. v.d., "Health systems across Europe; similarities and differences", WHO regional office for Europe, Copenhagen, 1992
60. Wyss, Marc, "Beschäftigte im Gesundheitswesen. Eine Analyse der Daten aus den Betriebszählungen von 1985 und 1991", Statistik der Schweiz, Gesundheit. Bern: Bundesamt für Statistik, 1993 / "Emplois dans le domaine de la santé. Une analyse des données des recensements des entreprises de 1985 et de 1991", Statistique de la Suisse, Santé. Berne: Office fédéral de la statistique, 1993.
61. Wyss, Marc et al., "Stationäre sozialmedizinische Institutionen. Ueberblick Schweiz und Kantone 1991", Statistik der Schweiz, Gesundheit. Bern: Bundesamt für Statistik, 1993 / "Etablissements de santé non hospitaliers. Un aperçu des résultats au niveau suisse et par canton 1991", Statistique de la Suisse, Santé. Berne: Office fédéral de la statistique, 1993.
62. Wyss, Marc, "Gesundheitsberufe in der Schweiz. Entwicklung von 1970 bis 1990", Eidgenössische Volkszählung 1990, Statistik der Schweiz, Gesundheit. Bern: Bundesamt für Statistik, 1995/"Professions de la santé en Suisse. Evolution de 1970 à 1990", Recensement fédéral de la population 1990, Statistique de la Suisse, Santé. Berne: Office fédéral de la statistique, 1995.
63. Zee, J. van der, "Home care in Denmark" in "Home care in Europe", edited by Hutten, J.B.F. and Jerkstra, A., p. 82–96, Aldershot, 1996.